Alkaline Protein Smoothies

Delicious & Nutritious, 100% Plant-Based Smoothie Recipes for a Super Healthy Lifestyle, Holistic Balance, and Natural Weight Loss

By Marta "Wellness" Tuchowska

All information in this book has been carefully researched and checked for factual accuracy. However, the author and publishers make no warranty, expressed or implied, that the information contained herein is appropriate for every individual, situation or purpose, and assume no responsibility for any errors or omissions.

The reader assumes the risk and full responsibility for all actions and the author will not be held liable for any loss or damage, whether consequential, incidental, and special or otherwise, that may result from the information presented in this publication.

The book is not intended to provide medical advice or to take the place of medical advice and treatment from your personal physician. Readers are advised to consult their own doctors or other qualified health professionals regarding the treatment of medical conditions.

The author shall not be held liable or responsible for any misunderstanding or misuse of the information contained in this book. The information is not intended to diagnose, treat or cure any disease.

Contents

Part 1: Introduction to the World of Alkaline Protein Smoothies

Thank you so much for taking an interest in this publication. I am very excited for you because the book you are holding in your hands has the potential to truly revolutionize your health and improve your wellbeing.

Alkaline protein smoothies are made of nutrient-dense, energy packed and balance stimulating vegetables, fruits, herbs, greens and super-healthy, hydrating liquids to help you create a new, more empowered version of yourself.

The best part? They are ridiculously easy to make, and this book will quickly guide you in the right direction so that you can become a true alkaline smoothie expert. Even if right now you are new to the world of smoothies, the alkaline diet and a healthy lifestyle, don't worry. I will take you by the hand and show you exactly what steps you need to take, so that you can focus on creating sustainable results without feeling overwhelmed.

If you are already a health veteran, I am positive you will discover new ways of spicing up your smoothie routine and gain some new, empowering information to help you reach new goals on your wellness quest.

This guide is written as a practical and easy to follow manual for a busy person who is health conscious, values their wellbeing but doesn't have the time for overcomplicating their wellness rituals or deciphering complicated information.

The good news is: Simplicity means wellness.
Alkaline protein smoothies truly hold the power to solve many
challenges and problems that people on the Alkaline Diet
lifestyle or any healthy lifestyle might have, such as:

- "I want to eat healthier, but I don't have the time to cook
healthy food all the time."

- "I tried smoothies. I really did my best but the ones I tried
didn't taste very good. Can I actually make a smoothie that
doesn't taste gross?"

- "I wanted to try a healthy lifestyle, but I was advised to buy
all those expensive powders and supplements. Is there a
simpler way to make healthy, alkaline smoothies?"

-"I really wanted to give this alkaline thing a try, but I didn't
know who to listen to and after doing some online research my
head was spinning. I am still not too sure which foods are
actually alkaline or what the point of this diet is."

- "I love smoothies, but, because of my health condition, I can't
have too much fruit because of the sugar it contains. Is there a
way to make vegetable smoothies taste nice?"

- "I like having a healthy lifestyle, but when I am stressed, I
tend to get off track, is there a way to increase my motivation?"

And so, on and so forth. But the good news is- you can put all
your worries and concerns away and allow yourself to discover
the new way of making delicious, satisfying, filling smoothies
in all flavors – sweet, spicy or natural.

The smoothie recipes I share in this book are rich in natural, plant-based protein that will help you stay full for hours. A proper alkaline protein smoothie for breakfast will help you stay full until lunch and avoid sugar temptations at work. It's not even about "staying full" as the main goal. The main goal is to stay nourished, energized and balanced. When that state of optimal wellness is achieved (and it's totally doable with alkaline protein smoothies and a healthy balanced lifestyle!), your body no longer lacks nutrients. Because of that it can pay you back with vibrant health and energy. You feel more focused and happier. When you give yourself permission to experience such a state, you actually crave more and more health and you truly enjoy healthy eating and conscious living.

Even a small serving of a nutrient and protein packed alkaline smoothie in the afternoon can help you feel more energized throughout the evening, so that you feel empowered to pursue your passions and spend quality time with your family, without dozing off on the couch. At the same time, you will be less likely to binge on unhealthy foods before dinner time, and when dinner is served, you will feel much more empowered to choose something healthy. Healthy choices attract more health.

Please note, this book, alkaline diet and alkaline protein smoothies are not only for vegans, vegetarians, alkaline-freaks or "plant-based-tarians". I truly welcome you all. Whatever diet you follow, I am confident you can add alkaline protein smoothies as a tool to your health and wellness toolbox.

Also, this book is not a strict diet book, nor a smoothie cleanse book. Be free to pick and choose the tips and recipes you feel can help you at the current stage of your journey. Focus on adding an abundance of nutrient-packed alkaline foods and drinks to your diet.

This mindset is so liberating, isn't it? Most diet books start off with, "Get rid of this, don't eat that." And yes, needless to say, to live a healthy lifestyle we need to let go of unhealthy habits. However, this is so much easier to achieve when we allow ourselves to focus on abundance first.

In this book, you'll find no bashing, no nutritional dogmas, no dietary religions, no shaming, no "holier-than-thou" attitudes. Nothing of that kind. We are in this together!

I myself had to overcome many physical, mental and emotional challenges which turned me into the person that I am today.

(I share my full story at the end of this book, for now I want to keep it short and sweet.)

This is how real transformation takes place- through overcoming challenges on a day-to-day basis. Nobody is perfect.

My role here is that of a messenger and someone who is with you in the trenches. I am simply sharing a very powerful wellness tool (alkaline protein smoothies) that you can incorporate into your lifestyle. I am not some ivory tower guru telling you what to do or trying to indoctrinate you into something without allowing you to think for yourself. You really need to be your own guru and tune into your body, mind and soul. You'll then be equipped to make choices that align with your health and wellness goals.

I have been living and teaching the Alkaline Diet and lifestyle for over five years now and it has truly helped me transform not only the way I eat, but also the way I live.

I am a self-care coach, and an author of numerous wellness books. I'm a certified holistic nutritionist, aromatherapist and reiki practitioner. I have been blessed to be able to study and practice many life-changing natural therapies and I love all of them, but the Alkaline Diet lifestyle is certainly one of my favorite tools to share and teach.

The reason I am so passionate about it is that it follows a truly holistic approach and helps your body restore the balance that it needs to create vibrant health and to heal on a deeper level. It also helps you feel amazing, not only physically but also emotionally. This will be a result of increasing your intake of nutrient rich foods and improving your energy levels. It's also flexible and can be successfully combined with other healthy diets that you may have found beneficial. Also, it doesn't require you to go on a crazy, restrictive diet where you are supposed to starve yourself.

That alone is so empowering! People around you will notice your shift and that healthy glow around you. They will want to know your secrets, trust me on that one.

Now, I really want to keep this book practical and to the point. It's not about me, it's about you and your journey.

So, here's the exact plan for this alkaline protein smoothie party:
1. First, I will guide you through the food lists and shopping lists so you can get started as soon as possible.

Aside from just listing the foods and ingredients you will need for making alkaline protein smoothies, I will be explaining different factors that determine whether a given ingredient is alkaline or not and how to create balance and nutritional abundance without becoming too strict with yourself.

2. Then, I will guide you through a very easy to understand and apply Alkaline Diet Crash Course. Everything will be very easy after the first step! It will make so much sense, that very soon you will be able to tell what is alkaline intuitively, without even checking the food lists. If a skeptical friend asks you about this diet, you will know what to say and get them interested in the alkaline way of living too.

3. Finally, I will show you how to use this book to make sure you create the results you deserve and feel inspired to take meaningful action towards your health goals, for years to come. It's not about "going on a diet" for a week or two. It's about creating sustainable balance for years to come and loving the process of who you are becoming.

Oh, and then we will get to the "meat and potatoes" of alkaline protein smoothies. With over fifty beautiful and inspiring recipes (plus a few bonus recipes), I am positive you will pick at least a few you can't wait to try and enjoy!

In this book, just like in my other books on the Alkaline Diet, healthy lifestyle, mindfulness and spiritual wellness, it's not only about giving you information. We also all need motivation and inspiration to stay on track and shift to vibrant health while enjoying our journey and inspiring those around us.

It is my deep intention that you use this booklet for years to come and discover how much positive change you can create by taking those little inspired courageous steps every day. My mission is to inspire people to eat, drink and live more alkaline so that they can create long-lasting transformation in all areas of their lives.

It all starts with health. Some people say, "Health is wealth." I agree, but I would say that health is more than that. Health is life. Value it, put it as your number one priority. Trust me, everything else will fall into place- your family, your career, your finances and your relationships. With vibrant health comes the courage and confidence to transform other areas of your life and live your true potential the way you were meant to.

Let's do this.

I love you; I appreciate you and I want to thank you once again for taking an interest in this publication and investing your precious time in learning with me.

We're in this together and I am looking forward to guiding you through this book. I am super-excited for you!

Marta "Wellness" Tuchowska

Alkaline Protein Smoothies- Food Lists

Recommended Alkaline Fruit

As a general rule, the Alkaline Diet encourages you to focus on fruits that are low in sugar. That is why the following fruits are considered super-alkaline:

- Lime
- Lemon
- Grapefruit
- Avocado (yes, it's a fruit)
- Tomato (yes, it's a fruit)
- Pomegranate

Yes, acidic-tasting lemons, limes and grapefruits are actually alkaline-forming fruits. The simplest explanation for it is that these fruits are very low in sugar and, at the same time, contain alkaline minerals such as Magnesium and Potassium.

So, to make strictly alkaline smoothies, we will focus more on using alkaline fruit. However, that doesn't mean you have to stay away from all the other types of fruit forever. Any fruit is a great addition to a healthy, balanced diet and makes your smoothies taste great.

When it comes to fruit, personally, I am somewhere in the middle of the road. I am not on the "avoid all fruit forever" bandwagon, just like I am not on the "eat endless amounts of bananas or be a fruitarian bandwagon". I have nothing against those, because people can choose how they want to eat. Everyone is different which is the beauty of life. But, personally, I am on the "follow yourself and listen to your body bandwagon."

It's all about balance!

That is why I focus a lot on strictly alkaline fruit (the fruit listed above), but I also listen to my body and go for other fresh, seasonal fruit as a part of a balanced diet.

This book will show you the art of strictly alkaline smoothies, as well as mixed, balanced, almost alkaline smoothies. The first 25 smoothie recipes in this book are "super-strictly" alkaline, while the rest are moderately alkaline.

If you need to follow a strict, low-sugar diet because of any medical condition, or a dietary choice (such as low carb or keto), or if your physician has recommended that you reduce all forms of sugar, then, needless to say it's recommended you focus on super-alkaline fruit (such as fruit low in sugar).

One thing is for sure, it's much better to have fruit than to binge on candy, processed sugar or processed carbs.
So, as a general rule- it's all about balance.

The following fruit is also great for moderate to neutral alkaline smoothies (although, these are not considered super-alkaline fruits because they are richer in sugar than the first list of fruit I shared above).
- Blueberries
- Sour cherries
- Raspberries
- Strawberries
- Other berries
- Green apples
- Watermelon
- Oranges

- Other fresh fruit to sweeten etc.

Greens

Greens are very good for you and are super-alkaline.
No worries, they will taste really nice in your smoothies. The recipes contained in this book have got you covered.

Greens to use in your smoothies:

- Spinach
- Kale
- Microgreens
- Swiss chard
- Arugula
- Endive
- Romaine lettuce

+ other fresh leafy greens and greens as well as herbs like:

- Parsley
- Mint
- Chives
- Dill

The goal of this book is to help you figure out what you like and what works for you.

Some people love spinach, while some prefer arugula or kale. It's not about forcing yourself to eat or drink something you absolutely can't stand. It's about mindfully exploring different options with the curiosity of a little child so that you can create a diet and lifestyle that you enjoy.

Do you need any green powders or supplements to make green or alkaline smoothies?

I always prefer fresh greens to green powders...but...whenever I go traveling, or I am really pressed for time, I like to use a green powder blend.

I also like to add it to my recipes as it makes my smoothies taste good while adding a ton of superfoods at the same time.

Other supplements and superfoods I like to use in my smoothies:
-Turmeric powder (very alkaline)
-Maca powder (natural hormone balancer)
-Ashwagandha powder (great for restoring balance, whether you need to calm down or create more energy)
-Moringa powder (very alkaline)

Alkaline Veggies

All fresh veggies are considered alkaline! So, this one is very easy. One of the goals of the alkaline diet is to encourage you to enrich your diet with more vegetables and greens. The real alkaline superfoods are very easy to find. Nature is all we need to restore vibrant health.

These are my favorite veggies to use in smoothies:

- Red bell pepper
- Green bell pepper
- Yellow bell pepper
- Zucchini (steamed, lightly cooked or raw)
- Broccoli (steamed, lightly cooked or raw)

- Asparagus (steamed, lightly cooked or raw)
- Cauliflower (steamed, lightly cooked or raw)
- Garlic
- Onion
- Cucumber
- Radish
- Artichoke (peeled and cooked)
- Carrot
- Sweet potato (peeled and cooked)

What I really love about using veggies in my smoothies is that they also allow me to create super-simple and satisfying creams and soups. These are great as a cleansing detox meal, or as a side dish to a "normal meal" to help add some nutrients and alkalinity.

Alkaline Spices & Herbs for Your Smoothies

The following herbs and spices will make your smoothies taste original, inspiring and truly delicious. They are also full of anti-inflammatory properties and can easily turn any smoothie into a truly unforgettable superfood smoothie:

- Cinnamon
- Himalayan salt
- Curry powder
- Red chili powder
- Cumin
- Nutmeg
- Italian herbs
- Oregano
- Rosemary

- Lavender
- Mint
- Chamomile
- Fennel
- Cilantro
- Stevia

The smoothie recipes from this book will give you guidelines on how to use some of the herbs mentioned above to create specific, therapeutic smoothies, such as an anti-insomnia smoothie, a relaxation smoothie and more.

Aside from helping you add more vitamins, minerals and natural protein to your diet, alkaline protein smoothies can help you feel more relaxed, sleep better and reduce some annoying symptoms such as PMS (pre-menstrual syndrome), digestive issues, or everyday stress (stress is very acidic).

Alkaline Sweeteners and Supplements (Optional)

- Stevia (it can be very helpful if you want to make a sweet smoothie without using sugar or sugar-containing foods or supplements)
- Green powders
- Moringa powder
- Maca powder
- Ashwagandha powder

I recommend you discuss using any supplement, even a natural one, with your doctor, especially if you are on medication (natural or allopathic), are pregnant or lactating, or suffering from any medical condition. Even if you are taking natural supplements at this stage, be sure to check for possible contraindications. Remember, supplements themselves will not help if your diet is not healthy and balanced. As the name suggests – supplements- just supplement.

Healthy Alkaline Oils to Add to Your Smoothies

- Olive oil (organic, cold-pressed)
- Avocado oil
- Hemp oil
- Flaxseed oil
- Coconut oil
- Sesame oil

Alkaline Nuts and Seeds

- Almonds (super-alkaline!)
- Cashews
- Brazil nuts
- Macadamia nuts
- Walnuts
- Pine nuts
- Pistachios
- Hazelnuts

These are also great natural sources of protein and good fats. The most alkaline nuts are almonds (almond milk is also great as we will soon find out). All nuts and seeds are a good addition to your smoothies, but be sure to buy only raw, natural, unsweetened, unsalted nuts and seeds. The reason for this is that processed nuts contain processed sugar and sodium as well as unhealthy, industrial vegetable oils and fats.

Alkaline Friendly Plant-Based Milk and Other Liquids to Use in Smoothies

As you may already know, dairy is not good for you, and so there is no dairy on the Alkaline Diet. (In this sense, the Alkaline Diet is similar to the Paleo Diet which also excludes milk and dairy products.)

Most people experience a significantly positive shift in their energy, wellbeing and vitality just by cutting out (or reducing) dairy from their diet.

For me personally, getting rid of dairy was a big game changer. I no longer get any nasty allergies, my digestion has improved, and I no longer feel that annoying burning inflammation in my stomach. Not to mention the fact that I get sick much less, and if I do, I recover very fast. Oh, and my skin is happy too!

I have been living a dairy free lifestyle for a few years now. Prior to that, on the first stage of my wellness journey, I studied the macrobiotic diet. I already knew for sure that dairy wasn't my best friend. However, at that time, there was still not that much information on the healthy, plant-based milk options available (aside from soy milk, which, according to the latest research, is not that good for us either).

Luckily, things have now changed, and more and more delicious and nutritious, fully plant-based, healthy milk variations are available even in mainstream supermarkets. Living a healthy lifestyle has never been easier so if you are only commencing on your journey now, you really should be grateful.

Super-Alkaline Plant-Based Milk
- Almond milk
- Coconut milk

Coconut and almond milk are highly alkalizing and nutrient-packed plant-based milk options. They are also good for alkaline detox or cleansing programs (more on that later). Some people are allergic to coconut and/or almond milk, or perhaps they don't like them for whatever reason.

If that's the case, there are other options available to help you make delicious plant-based smoothies.

Other alkaline liquids to use in your smoothies include:
-all kinds of herbal infusions (caffeine-free)
-coconut water (no added sugar)
-clean, filtered, alkaline water

You can also use other plant-based milk such as:
-cashew milk
-gluten-free oat milk
-hazelnut milk
-quinoa milk

These are less alkaline than coconut and almond milk (a staple plant-based milk on the alkaline diet) but are still healthy and nutritious.

My favorites are definitely coconut and almond milk (very alkaline, as well as paleo and keto friendly) but sometimes I also like to use some oat milk or other delicious, creamy plant-based milk for more variety.

Just be sure to go for unsweetened, all-natural options with no processed vegetable oils added. (The addition of Himalayan salt is fine.)

The bottom line is- stay away from dairy, and experiment with different plant-based milk options to before choosing what works best for you.

Plant-Based Clean Protein Sources to Use in Your Alkaline Smoothies

- Hemp seeds and hemp seed powder
- Chia seeds and chia seed powder
- Almonds, almond powder and almond milk
- Organic, gluten-free oats and oat milk
- Quinoa (cooked)
- Pumpkin seeds
- Pistachios
- Flax seeds
- Sesame seeds
- Fresh, raw nut butters (for example, almond or cashew)
- Dark, green veggies (for example, kale and spinach)

Now, it's time for a bit of simple theory.

The hardest part is already behind you because now you understand what alkaline foods look like. So, the next section should be enjoyable and easy to digest. (Alkaline books should be easy to digest, otherwise they are not so alkaline!)

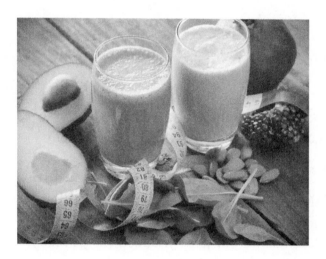

The Alkaline Diet Beginner-Friendly Crash Course

I am sure you have been waiting for this! Since the book has the word "Alkaline" in the title, I am sure you have been expecting me to write a little bit about the pH.

The good news is that it's not as complicated as many gurus want us to believe. In fact, it's pretty common sense, healthy eating knowledge.

The pH of most of our crucial cellular and other body fluids, like blood, is designed to be at a pH of 7.365 which is slightly alkaline.

Luckily, our miraculous body has an intricate system in place to maintain that healthy, slightly alkaline pH level. It's working for us 24/7, to ensure our pH system stays optimally balanced.

An interesting thing is that our body, as long as it is blessed with the gift of life, will continuously keep working to regulate our pH (whether we eat a healthy diet rich in alkaline foods or not).

The problem? It's up to us to make it easier or harder for our body...

We can totally choose what we eat. But...if we focus on unhealthy choices, for example the Standard Western Diet with its overload of sugars, processed carbohydrates, dairy, soda, too many animal products, and fast food we make it more and more difficult for our body to stay in balance. Some people say, "Oh, but what is the point of eating a healthy diet rich in alkaline unprocessed foods if our body regulates our pH for us?"

Yes, our body regulates our pH for us, no matter what we eat. We can't make our pH higher and higher. You see, this is not the goal of the alkaline diet. We just can't make our blood's pH more alkaline or "higher." Our body tries to work hard for us to help maintain our ideal pH. We can't have a pH of 8 or 9. It's not about magically raising or re-modifying our body's pH level.

The focus of the alkaline diet is to give your body the nourishment and the healing tools that it needs to MAINTAIN that optimal pH almost effortlessly.

This is achieved by taking in healthy, balanced nutrition rich in alkaline foods (you already know these are good for you!) such as:
- unprocessed foods
- naturally gluten-free foods
- yeast-free foods
- dairy-free foods
- sugar-free foods
- wheat-free foods
- foods rich in minerals, vitamins and chlorophyll
-plant-based foods, greens and veggies

If we do not support our bodies with healthy, balanced nutrition, we torture them with incredible stress! Yes, when the body has to continually work overtime to detoxify all of the cells and maintain our pH, it finally succumbs to disease. It

27

still keeps working and balancing...but...it gets weaker and weaker and we no longer get to enjoy the vibrant health and vitality of our dreams. This is when we become much more prone to disease and there's a downward spiral of physical and mental ailments.

Let me give a few examples of what can happen if we continuously eat an acid-forming diet (also called SAD - Standard American Diet, or Standard Western Diet) that does not support our body at all. Our body ends up sick and tired of working overtime and may manifest one or more of the following conditions:

- Chronic inflammation
- Immune and hormonal imbalance
- Lack of energy, mental fog- you go for another cup of coffee yet still feel the same, sound familiar?
- Yeast and candida overgrowth
- Digestive damage
- Weakened bones. Our body is forced to pull minerals <u>like magnesium and calcium from our bones to maintain the alkaline balance it needs for constant healing processes.</u>

In summary, eating more alkaline foods, for example veggies, herbs, and greens, helps support our body so that it can work for us at optimal levels. Eating more acidic foods (aka processed food, fast food, sugar, soda, too many animal products etc.) doesn't help at all. The alkaline diet is not about magically raising or changing our pH, but about helping our body rebalance itself by supporting its natural healing functions with healthy food and drink such as alkaline smoothies.

The commonsense explanation is to imagine you eat a hardcore Western Diet for a month. You eat processed carbs, fast food, drink soda and bombard your body with unhealthy fats, sugars and way too many animal products. You don't drink enough water and you don't move your body. Needless to say, your wellbeing will not improve, and you will begin to feel tired and will very likely have pain and inflammation. (Fair enough, if you are very young, it may take some time to develop those unhealthy symptoms, but why do that to yourself?)

Then, imagine that you focus on a clean food diet (whether it's fully plant-based, or almost plant-based). You eat lots of vegetables, whole foods and unprocessed foods. In other words, you eat a diet rich in alkaline foods. You also drink lots of clean water and nutrient packed smoothies with healthy alkaline vegetables and fruit. Yes, fair enough, every now and then, you have a treat meal or indulge in acidity very occasionally. However, your overall healthy balance is so strong that your body copes well.

Needless to say, by eating better, by eating a clean food diet and optimizing your health, you feel better and allow your body to heal faster. You treat your body as a temple!

For example, our body also regulates our temperature for us. But...what will happen if you immerse yourself in a bath full of ice cubes for too long? How long will your body keep going and regulate your temperature for you? Everything has a limit. We can only rely on our "health credit cards" for so long...The first step for most people is to pay off that "health debt". The second step is to make sure your alkaline bank account still has funds in it. The third step is to embrace the Health Investor mindset. Every food choice we make can be an

investment, or an asset, for our long-term wellness, or it can be a distraction. The question I ask myself every day is: *Am I getting closer to or farther away from my vision?*
The Alkaline Diet is sisters with the Clean Food Diet, Anti-Inflammatory Diet, Vegetarian Diet, Vegan Diet, Macrobiotic Diet, and the Raw Food Diet. In fact, it offers an incredible blend and the best of them all. All those diets that are more in the plant-based category.

However, what may come as a big surprise to many is that there are also many similarities with Keto and Paleo Diets. Similarly to a Paleo Diet (Paleolithic Diet), the Alkaline Diet encourages you to stay away from dairy and wheat as well as processed carbs (such as pasta).

Similarly to the Keto Diet, the Alkaline Diet loves good fats (predominantly in their plant-based version). Also, when it comes to fruit, it encourages you to focus mostly on low-sugar fruit (as we have already covered in the first section of alkaline food lists).

Oh, and again - no nasty, processed carbs. (The Alkaline Diet encourages natural, unprocessed sources of good, healthy carbohydrates that will help you thrive!)

That is why the Alkaline Diet is not just a diet. It's a lifestyle. A nutritionally reasonable, healthily flexible lifestyle that can be combined with other diets you already like and benefit from to make them work even better for you. (Yes, there is Alkaline Plant-Based, Alkaline Almost Plant-Based, Alkaline Vegetarian, Alkaline Paleo, Alkaline Keto, Alkaline Mediterranean etc.).

THE ALKALINE CRASH COURSE

Different strokes for different folks. However, the healthy foundation remains the same: add a ton of alkaline foods into your diet. It's an investment in your health and wellbeing.

What do all the alkaline foods and drinks have in common?

This one is one of my favorite questions. The answer below will help you reverse-engineer different foods to determine whether they are alkaline or not.

As a general rule, all alkaline foods and drinks are naturally

- low in sugar
- gluten-free
- dairy-free
- yeast-free
- high in nutrients (vitamins and minerals)
- plant-based (when going alkaline, you can do a fully plant-based alkaline diet, or reduce your intake of animal products while massively increasing the intake of plant-based foods)
- alcohol-free and caffeine free (no worries, as long as you help your body stay in balance and you eat and drink healthily, you can enjoy a glass of wine or a cup of coffee as an occasional treat).
- green -unless they contain caffeine or are high in sugar. For example, green tea is not so alkaline.

(I still use it every now and then.)

Matcha tea isn't, either.

(Again, I still occasionally use it as a non-alkaline part of my diet).

31

Kiwi fruit aren't very alkaline but every now and then I use them in my smoothies or snack on them.

There are many healthy foods and superfoods that are not considered alkaline, and that's OK. The point of the Alkaline Diet (as you will soon find out, or maybe you already know) isn't to eat 100% alkaline all the time. This brings us to the next question...

Isn't it hard to eat alkaline all the time? I like the sound of the health benefits and all that, but I don't think I can eat that way all the time.

The reason I love the Alkaline Diet and have been able to live this lifestyle for over 5 years (and I really enjoy it, lost weight, feel good and all that) is because of the alkaline 80/20 rule that most alkaline experts recommend. (It works so well!)

The rule is very simple. Your goal should be to make about 80% of your diet alkaline, while the remaining 20% can be other foods. Even 70/30 is a great start for most people.

It's as simple as making about three quarters of your plate full of alkaline foods, for example veggies. That allows for some flexibility as well as respect for other nutritional choices you may wish to combine with the Alkaline Diet.

Of course, it's all about common sense...The 80/20 rule should not be interpreted as an 80% super-strict, crazy alkaline regime and 20% eat-whatever-you-want, no limits, fast food, processed junk food.

That would only confuse your body and spoil all the health and wellness efforts you have worked so hard for.

To live this rule with optimum benefit and maximum pleasure, the most reasonable and common-sense thing to do is this:

- Focus about 80% of your diet and lifestyle on delicious alkaline-friendly foods and drinks (fresh salads, more vegetables, yummy soups, satisfying warm alkaline meals, smoothies, greens, juices...all the good stuff).

You can get started step-by-step, absolutely pain-free by combining alkaline foods with "normal food". For example, add a salad to your regular meal. Alternatively, make a delicious smoothie for breakfast. Start with small goals. Focus first on adding things, focus on abundance.

- Then, for the rest of your diet (about 20%)- add other foods you feel that your body needs. These may not necessarily be super-alkaline foods, but should still be clean, unprocessed foods as far as possible, including traditional home cooked meals you like. Within that 20%, a small percentage can be a *now-and-then-indulge-in-some-acidity* treat.

Personally, I love to keep this treat for social occasions and family gatherings. At times like this, I will still drink lots of water, add my alkaline smoothies and alkaline juices and take care of what I like to call "My healthy alkaline foundation". But...on a special occasion, I will also enjoy a family meal out without worrying all the time about what I eat, or feeling like an alien. I will order my favorite meal with a big bowl of salad, enjoy my time out with family and friends and the next morning will proceed to make myself a massive alkaline smoothie. Business as usual!

The most important thing is to focus on balance and listen to your body. My goal behind writing this book is to simply

inspire you to enrich your diet and lifestyle with alkaline foods and drinks. Oh, and alkaline emotions too...
You see, the Alkaline Diet lifestyle is not only about what you eat, but it's also about how you live...

Stress is very acid-forming and unfortunately in this day and age it's so easy to feel stressed.

Aside from having demanding professional work and family obligations, bills to pay, goals to achieve etc. we may get over-exposed to social media and online advertisements. Not only do we spend more and more time on our computers and mobile devices, but we may also get exposed to some negative messaging while online or watching TV. Messages that tell us, for instance, that we are not slim, rich, happy, loved and fit enough, so we must be doing something wrong...)

The messages and advertisements we get exposed to are very often fear-based and designed to make us feel bad about ourselves. We feel as if we are not good enough.

Our mind can easily get on a downward spiral of negative emotions. By default, we become conditioned to focus on the negative. We feel guilty and allow someone to shame us and bash us. That makes us separate from our true self, our inner guidance and inner light that wants us to be healthy.

Fortunately, we also live in very interesting times when more and more people are seeking empowerment and positive information through loved-based actions and choices. As a writer, I feel incredibly blessed to be on the loved-based messaging "bandwagon" to inspire people and hopefully help them make changes in alignment with their personal choices and lifestyle, without interfering with their inner peace and their personal journey. (Our journeys get shaped by a myriad of different factors and experiences that are unique to us- it's not only about what we eat, diet is merely one of the factors we can use to create holistic wellness.)

Loved-based and fear-based concepts can also be observed in everyday life. When you have a look at all the good decisions you have made, you will probably conclude that they came from love, not from fear.

I always say that it's all about acting from a place of wholeness, confidence and abundance. Allow yourself to feel whole and complete right here right now. Love your body the way it is. Stop torturing yourself with negative thoughts.

Focus on the positive. Take positive action. Love yourself the way you are and never beat yourself up. Respect yourself and your journey. Negative emotions can get us off track. Life can get in the way as things happen. It's normal to experience negative emotions as well. Nobody is perfect and in life we get to experience both positivity as well as negativity.

It's up to us to decide what we focus on. Do not allow anyone make you feel bad about yourself with their fear-based, manipulative messaging. Be yourself, think for yourself, choose for yourself.

You can choose to spend more time in nature instead of staying indoors in front of some screen with negative messaging on it. You can choose to read books written by loved-based authors, and you can watch videos that uplift you. You can choose to control your focus.

Ok, enough of my philosophical essays. You are probably thinking, "Hey, just give me those 50 alkaline smoothie recipes already please!"

The number one take-away from this section is this: focus on love and kindness as much as you can. That kindness starts with how you treat yourself and who you allow into your mind.

Exploring my mindset and my inner world has been helpful for me and has changed my relationship with food and helped me stay healthy. I truly believe in mind-body power and in the healing power of love and positive emotions.

Now back to foods...

What is the difference between the alkaline cleanse and alkaline lifestyle? Do I need to eat this way all the time?

I have noticed that many Alkaline Diet beginners get a bit stuck or confused here and this prevents them from taking action.

Luckily, it's not that complicated. The Alkaline Diet lifestyle is a simple, balanced, clean food diet combining a healthy lifestyle enriched with a ton of fresh alkaline foods.

It's all about progress, not about being perfect, and it's not about eating 100% alkaline. (Honestly, I don't know anyone who eats 100% alkaline all the time.)

The basic rule is to focus on an abundance of fresh foods, especially veggies, greens and low sugar fruit. On the Alkaline

Diet lifestyle, as you already know, you aim to make about 70-80% of your diet rich in alkaline foods, while the remaining 20-30% can be other foods. Still, these should not be processed fast foods. You should still aim for quality, clean food, so that at least even if it's not alkaline, it's still healthy food.

It's all about balance here.

With such a healthy foundation, it's okay to have some treats here and there, like a coffee, a glass of wine, or your favorite foods on a family occasion or social get together.

The Alkaline Diet lifestyle can be either fully plant-based, if you want, or it can be combined with other diets, for example, Paleo or Mediterranean.

It's very flexible and if you already have another healthy diet that you follow, you can always benefit from enriching your existing diet with more fresh, alkaline foods. This can be done with salads, soups, smoothies, juices, or adding more veggies to your "normal food". That sums up pretty much everything I teach through my books and programs -balance.

However, in some circumstances you may also benefit from doing an alkaline cleanse...

Ok, so what is an alkaline cleanse? Do I do it?

Yes, 2-3 times a year, I like to go fully alkaline for a week or two with a goal of restoring my energy, getting rid of toxins, and giving my body, mind and soul a "break".

Alkaline Cleanse – this is basically when you go fully alkaline for certain period of time, usually a week or two, with an intention of deep healing. It may also be a wonderful solution for those who really need a strong dose of alkalinity to bring their bodies back into balance.

As always, before going on any kind of cleanse, I advise you to consult with your doctor, especially if you are on any medication or experiencing any serious health issues.

Whenever I go on an alkaline cleanse, I nourish myself with 100% alkaline meals, drinks, tonics and I also drink lots of alkaline juice and smoothies. Yes, I eat 100% alkaline for a week or two (with a little preparation period and after the cleanse period).

During this time, I have no processed foods and no caffeine. This can be a bit difficult if you are hooked on caffeine, but totally worth it, because the energy you will get after the cleanse is truly amazing! I also have no alcohol. No acidic foods at all. No sugar. Only 100% alkaline plant-based foods.

And a lot of rest while doing this.

Now, while it may sound a bit challenging, for many people an alkaline cleanse is actually an amazing experience when done properly (enough calories and macros per day etc.) by following delicious recipes and guidelines. It's not just about doing some fad cleanse or a weird one-ingredient detox cleanse. It's about using a variety of different recipes that are 100% alkaline and that help your body restore all its systems. Every time I do an alkaline cleanse, I feel stronger, not only physically but also mentally and emotionally and my nutritional and lifestyle choices get better and better.

After the cleanse my habits always improve, and I learn a lot about myself and my relationship with food. It feels so good to use food positively as a tool to nourish myself. I feel free to break away from patterns and cravings that do not serve my long-term vision.

As one of my health mentors, Yuri Elkaim says, "You crave what's in your blood."

So true! Plus, we can experience this state in both a negative and positive way. A healthy body surely craves more health. In some cases, to reach such a state, a proper alkaline cleanse is desperately needed.

You will notice that the recipes in this book are divided into two parts. The first part of the book will show you delicious, 100% alkaline recipes (compatible with alkaline cleanses), while the recipes from the second part of the book follow an 80/20 rule. They are rich in alkaline foods but also use other ingredients. This makes them what I like to call "almost alkaline", or "balanced" smoothies.

So, this book will be useful for you both if you are planning some kind of an alkaline detox, as well as for a healthy, balanced, alkaline lifestyle.

The topic of alkaline cleanses goes beyond the scope of this book. To learn more about cleansing, I recommend you read the book: *Alkaline Reset Cleanse* by Ross Bridgeford.

(Wow, that was quite an intro. By now you should have a better intuitive understanding of the Alkaline Diet and all you need to know to get started on alkaline protein smoothies.)

Alkaline Protein Smoothies- How to Use This Book

If you have any health conditions or allergies, be sure to double check with your doctor before starting. Get the full list of foods and ingredients you can't consume or are allergic too. Then, when going through this guide, you will be able to focus only on the recipes that don't use those ingredients, or use any recipe you want but entirely skip the ingredients you can't have or replace them.

In most cases, skipping one or two ingredients in a recipe will not make a huge difference, unless we are talking about crucial components of the recipes, in which case you will need to replace that ingredient with something similar. For example, coconut milk can be replaced with almond milk or any plant-based milk, or even water. Grapefruit can be replaced with lemons. Kale can be replaced with spinach.

It's all about creativity and flexibility.

Oh, and if you are new to some superfood like chia seeds, moringa powder etc, most of those can be easily found online. I buy most of mine via Amazon. It's easy and fast.

One of the best ways to embrace this lifestyle is to focus on adding more alkaline smoothies into your diet.

While most diets focus on counting calories and being restrictive, the Alkaline Diet focuses on abundance and on enriching your diet with nutrient-rich alkaline foods.

As soon as you focus on that and get rid of the *I need to be perfect* mindset, you will start creating amazing long-term results, like having more energy, and feeling happy and vibrant.

I highly recommend that you set a goal of having one massive alkaline protein smoothie a day. At the same time, reduce caffeine, drink plenty of fresh water, focus on eating clean and you will soon start experiencing the miracle of a simple, healthy lifestyle.

If you are new to this lifestyle, you may start off with this little template:

1. Morning- lots of water (or lemon water), herbal infusion (if you really need caffeine, use a bit of green tea) + big alkaline protein smoothie (make two servings and save one for the afternoon).
2. Mid-afternoon snack – some alkaline snack, like raw almonds, or celery sticks with humus and herbal infusion. You can also go for one serving of fresh, seasonal fruit.

3. Lunch- one big alkaline salad + something you would normally have (keep it as clean as possible and ban fast food and processed junk).

4. Afternoon snack – your smoothie.

5. Optional (I do it a few times a week) – make a big alkaline juice to enjoy one serving of fresh alkaline juice in the afternoon. It will give you more energy than coffee. Store the rest in the fridge to enjoy another serving the next morning. It's a great way to kick-start your morning. To learn more about alkaline juicing, you can explore my other book *Alkaline Juicing*.

6. Dinner- you can have something you would normally make plus a big plate of salad or veggies. Alternatively, you can make a delicious plant-based meal, or a meal rich in alkaline foods, to enjoy for dinner and lunch for the next day (whenever I cook, I cook in batches).

If you struggle to put veggies together and make them taste nice, I recommend you explore my other books such as : *Alkaline Salads*, or *Plant-Based Cookbook* for more ideas, outside of smoothies. Even a simple habit of serving your "normal meals" with a big plate of salads is a great way of moving forward, step-by-step!

At the same time, drink lots of clean, filtered water. Set a timer on your phone if you forget to drink water or link drinking water to another habit. I usually work in 1 hour or 45-minute blocks. So, when my timer goes off, I drink a glass of water. That easily allows me to get at least 1 liter of water (or more, because I also drink lots of water as a part of my morning ritual), in the early morning.

Important

1.*This is a simple to follow recipe and lifestyle book to inspire and motivate you on your wellness quest. However, it is not meant to diagnose or treat any medical conditions.*

If you are suffering from any chronic disease, have recently undergone any medical treatment, are pregnant, lactating or suffering from any serious health condition, you need to speak to your doctor first.

It is also recommended that you familiarize yourself with all the precautions that the extended use of certain herbs entails. Some herbs may interfere with certain medications, so if you take any, be sure to seek professional medical advice first.

2.*The book should also not be interpreted as a quick weight loss fad program. There is no secret sauce to losing weight. It's a journey that is different for different people (depending on their genetics, where they are coming from, their current habits, mindset, diet and many other factors and patterns). Natural and sustainable weight loss is achieved when you focus on health and balance and give your body what it needs to thrive. This book is a tool that can inspire you to live in alignment with that philosophy and help your body get back to its optimal, healthiest weight.*

Measurements Used in the Recipes

The cup measurement I use is the American Cup measurement.

I also use it for dry ingredients. If you are new to it, let me help you:

If you don't have American Cup measures, just use a metric or imperial liquid measuring jug and fill your jug with your ingredient to the corresponding level. Here's how to go about it:

1 American Cup= 250ml= 8 fl.oz.
For example:
If a recipe calls for 1 cup of almonds, simply place your almonds into your measuring jug until it reaches the 250 ml/8oz mark.

Quite easy, right?

I know that different countries use different measurements and I wanted to make things simple for you. I have also noticed that very often those who are used to American Cup measurements complain about metric measurements and vice versa. However, if you apply what I have just explained, you will find it easy to use both.

The Following Recipe Section (Recipes 1- 25) Contains 100% Alkaline Smoothie Recipes That Are Also Alkaline Detox Friendly.

Recipe #1 Creamy Alkaline Keto Energizer

This delicious smoothie combines greens with natural protein and good fats. Ginger adds to its anti-inflammatory properties and helps stimulate the lymphatic system. Maca is a natural energy booster and hormone rebalancer. The smoothie is naturally creamy and very tasty. The cinnamon powder really spices it up.

It's perfect for a busy day, when you need a ton of energy. This smoothie will help you create focus and thanks to its generous content of good, healthy fats, will help prevent sugar cravings.

Serves: 1-2
Ingredients
- Half cup fresh spinach leaves, washed
- 1 small avocado, peeled and pitted
- A handful of almonds, raw, soaked in filtered water for at least a few hours
- 1 tablespoon chia seeds
- 2 cups cold coconut milk, unsweetened
- 1 tablespoon coconut oil
- Half teaspoon maca
- 1 teaspoon cinnamon powder
- 2-inches fresh ginger, peeled
- Optional- stevia to sweeten

Instructions
1. Place all the ingredients in the blender.
2. Process until smooth.
3. Serve and enjoy! This nutritious smoothie makes a great breakfast.

Recipe #2 Creamy Protein Delight

This is one of my favorite super alkaline smoothies. It combines natural protein from chia seeds with good fats from avocado.

It's naturally creamy and beginner-friendly. Lemons (or limes) blend really well with avocados. This smoothie tastes a bit like Greek yoghurt but is fully plant-based and dairy free.

You can also serve this smoothie as a smoothie bowl, with some nuts and seeds (for example almonds and cashews).

Serves: 1-2

Ingredients
- 2 cups cold unsweetened coconut milk or almond milk
- 2 tablespoons chia seeds (or chia seed powder)
- 1 small lemon, peeled and sliced
- 1 small avocado, peeled and pitted
- a few lime slices to garnish
- a pinch of Himalayan salt

Instructions
1. Place all the ingredients in a blender.
2. Blend until smooth.
3. Pour into a smoothie glass, or serve in a small bowl with some nuts and seeds.
4. Enjoy!

Recipe #3 Beautiful Skin Alkaline Protein Drink

People always ask me about natural beauty tips and the Alkaline Diet can surely help! My recommendation is to focus on what you eat (and drink) first.

In my twenties (especially my early twenties) I spent lots of money on magic solutions, creams and other shortcuts. However, it was only when I decided to take care of the inside and put my health first that the real transformation took place.

This is one of my favorite 100% alkaline smoothie recipes that combines the power of beta-carotene rich ingredients to help you have beautiful, healthy looking skin.

This smoothie is also very filling and nourishing! Oh, and needless to say it tastes creamy. I am not a big fan of those pitiful smoothies that taste like baby food and take lots of willpower to get through as well.

Serves: 1-2
Ingredients
- 1 cup coconut or almond milk
- Half cup coconut water
- 2 small carrots, peeled
- 1 big red bell pepper, cut into smaller pieces
- 2 tablespoons hemp seed protein powder
- 1 teaspoon cinnamon powder

Optional- stevia to sweeten if needed
Optional- fresh mint leaves and lime slices to serve

Instructions

1. Place all the ingredients in a blender.
2. Blend until smooth.
3. Pour into a glass and enjoy!

This smoothie is a fantastic way of adding more veggies to your diet, first thing in the morning.

Red bell peppers are one of my favorite alkaline superfoods. They are naturally sweet, inexpensive and very easy to find (even in your local grocery store).

No excuses- a healthy lifestyle doesn't have to be about overpriced supplements and complicated rituals.

Creating a healthy foundation is all about simplicity, and what you need is already within your reach.

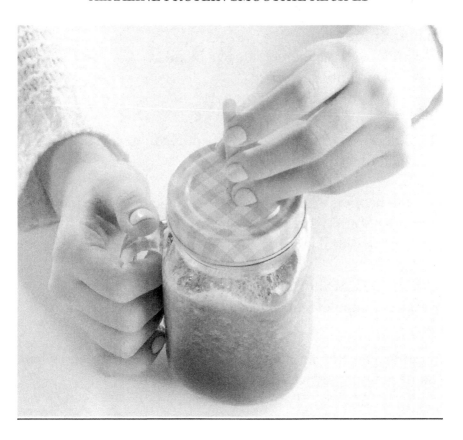

Recipe #4 Green Aroma Smoothie

Moringa is an alkaline superfood. It contains all the essential amino acids – the building blocks of protein- that are needed to grow, repair and maintain cells. At the same time, it's rich in alkaline forming minerals such as magnesium, iron and potassium.

Mint and cilantro give this smoothie a refreshing taste while adding a ton of micronutrients and antioxidants. They also aid in digestion. Perhaps you are not a big fan of spinach or kale smoothies, or maybe you are looking for new, original recipes. Well, the good news is that there are different options out there!

Serves: 1-2
Ingredients
- 1 cup almond milk
- A handful almonds, soaked in filtered water for at least a few hours
- 1 inch fresh ginger, peeled
- 1 teaspoon moringa powder
- A few avocado slices
- A handful fresh mint, washed
- A handful fresh cilantro leaves, washed

Instructions
1. Place all the ingredients into a blender
2. Process well until smooth.
3. Enjoy!

Recipe #5 Lime Flavored Protein Smoothie

This smoothie is great as a quick energizing snack or even as a dessert. It uses stevia to create natural sweetness. It's also rich in healthy protein, good fats and vitamin C. Cinnamon and ginger add to its alkaline and anti-inflammatory properties.

Serves: 1-2
Ingredients
- 1 cup unsweetened coconut or almond milk
- 2 small limes, peeled and cut into smaller pieces
- 1 teaspoon cinnamon powder
- 1-inch ginger, peeled
- 1 tablespoon avocado oil
- 1 tablespoon chia seeds
- Optional: stevia to sweeten

Instructions
1. Place all the ingredients in a blender.
2. Process well until smooth.
3. If needed, sweeten with stevia.

Serve in a smoothie glass and sprinkle some cinnamon powder on top for extra sweetness.

Recipe #6 Full-on Energy Alkaline Goodness

This smoothie combines spinach and grapefruits to help you enjoy more energy. Spinach is naturally rich in iron, and the vitamin C from grapefruits helps the body absorb it better.

Grapefruits also give this smoothie a refreshing flavor. Grapefruit, just like limes and lemons, is considered an alkaline-forming fruit because of its very low sugar content and high alkaline mineral profile.

Serves: 1-2
Ingredients
- 1 small avocado, peeled, pitted and sliced
- Half cup fresh spinach leaves, washed
- 1 big grapefruit, peeled and cut into smaller pieces
- 2 cups coconut water
- 2 tablespoons sunflower seeds

Instructions
1. Place all the ingredients in a blender.
2. Process well until smooth.
3. Coconut water should make this smoothie taste naturally sweet, however, if you need to, you can also add some stevia.

Recipe #7 Mediterranean Refreshment Smoothie

This recipe is similar to the original Spanish gazpacho recipe; however, it also sneaks in some greens, healthy fats and alkaline friendly protein.

It's so refreshing, jam packed with all the super nutrients and, thanks to a generous dose of Mediterranean herbs- wonderfully tasty and aromatic.

This smoothie can also be served as a delicious raw soup which makes it a great, nutritionally balanced, refreshing, super-healthy meal on a hot summer day. It could also be served as an appetizer, or combined with "normal food", unless you are cleansing.

Serves: 2-3
Ingredients
- 3 big tomatoes, roughly chopped
- 2 big cucumbers, peeled
- 2 slices of lime, peel removed
- 5 small radishes
- 1 big green bell pepper, roughly chopped
- A few onion rings
- 2 garlic cloves, peeled
- 2 cups water, filtered, preferably alkaline
- Half cup almond milk
- A handful of almonds, soaked in water for at least a few hours
- 2 tablespoons extra virgin, organic olive oil
- 2 generous pinches Himalayan salt
- Half teaspoon oregano

- Half teaspoon black pepper
- Half teaspoon basil (or a few fresh basil leaves)
- Half teaspoon parsley (or a few fresh parsley leaves)

To serve:
- 1-2 tablespoons fresh lemon juice to serve
- 1-2 tablespoons chopped chive to serve

Please note- this is a pretty long ingredient list, but don't worry about being too perfect. You can skip a couple of ingredients, and as you use this recipe several times, you will surely discover your favorite variations.

Instructions
1. Place all the ingredients in a blender.
2. Process well until smooth.
3. Taste to see if you need to add any more herbs, spices or Himalayan salt.
4. Serve in a small soup bowl, sprinkle over some fresh chive and lemon juice and enjoy this alkaline Mediterranean goodness!

Recipe #8 Easy White Chia Pick Me Up

I came up with this recipe by accident. I had run out of all my fruits and veggies (happens very often as I am a real smoothie and juice monster) except one little lime.

So, I decided to be proactive and blend a few simple, alkaline ingredients I had at hand. The result was amazing!

Serves: 1-2
Ingredients
- 1 lime, peeled and cut into smaller pieces
- 1 cup coconut milk, unsweetened
- 1 tablespoon chia seeds
- Half teaspoon cinnamon powder
- 1 generous pinch of nutmeg powder

Optional: stevia to sweeten

Instructions
1. Place all the ingredients in a blender.
2. Process until smooth.
3. Now, try the smoothie to see if you like the taste.
4. If needed, add in some stevia and blend again.
5. Place in a smoothie glass, drink and enjoy!

Recipe #9 Oriental Taste Cilantro Smoothie

This smoothie is spicy, nourishing, comforting and filling. It makes a truly delicious lunch smoothie recipe and can also be turned into a soup (raw or lightly cooked).

Sweet potatoes are a healthy source of good carbohydrates and they also make smoothies taste great. They are quick and easy to cook, and you could also use some dinner leftovers.

Serves: 2
Ingredients
- 2 sweet potatoes, peeled and cooked
- 1 big tomato, cut into smaller pieces
- A big handful of fresh cilantro leaves, washed
- A big handful of fresh parsley leaves, washed
- A few onion rings
- 1 big garlic clove, peeled
- 1-inch turmeric, peeled (use gloves unless you want to end up with naturally orange fingers and nails for a couple of days)
- 1 cup coconut milk
- 1 cup water, filtered, preferably alkaline
- 2 tablespoons raw almonds, soaked in water for at least a few hours
- A generous pinch of Himalayan salt
- A pinch red chili powder
- A pinch cumin powder
- A pinch black pepper powder
- 1 tablespoon extra-virgin, organic olive oil or avocado oil (cold pressed)
- 1 tablespoon lime juice, to serve

Instructions

1. Place all the ingredients in a blender.
2. Process until smooth.
3. Try the smoothie to see if you need to add more spices.
4. If needed, add more spices or Himalayan salt to taste.
5. Serve in a big smoothie glass, or a soup bowl.
6. Sprinkle over some lime juice and enjoy!

Recipe #10 Quinoa Protein Mineral Smoothie

Quinoa makes this smoothie super-filling and adds some natural protein. Cucumber and cilantro provide a ton of nutrients and minerals as well as an unforgettable, soft, refreshing taste.

This smoothie makes a great lunch and will help you stay energized throughout the whole afternoon.

Serves: 1-2

Ingredients

- 5 big tablespoons of quinoa, cooked and cooled down
- 1 big cucumber, peeled and cut into smaller pieces
- A big handful of cilantro leaves, washed
- 1 small garlic clove, peeled
- 1 cup coconut milk, unsweetened
- A pinch of Himalayan salt
- A pinch of cumin powder
- A pinch of curry powder
- A pinch of black pepper powder
- A wedge of lime, to serve

Instructions

1. Place all the ingredients in a blender.
2. Process well until smooth.
3. Serve as a smoothie or as a raw smoothie soup, and squeeze in some fresh lime juice.
4. Enjoy!

Recipe #11 Easy Green Protein Delight

Arugula is one of my favorite greens and it tastes fantastic in smoothies. It's very rich in calcium and iron as well as vitamin A. In this recipe, it blends well with herbs and spices to help you enjoy a highly alkaline green protein smoothie.

Serves: 1-2
Ingredients
- 1 cup fresh arugula leaves, washed
- A handful of fresh parsley leaves, washed
- A handful of cilantro leaves, washed
- A few lime slices, peeled
- 1 cup coconut milk
- 1 tablespoon chia seeds or chia seed powder
- A pinch of Himalayan salt
- A pinch of chili powder
- A pinch of black pepper powder
- A pinch of oregano

Instructions
1. Place all the ingredients in a blender.
2. Blend well until smooth.
3. Serve in a smoothie glass and enjoy!

Recipe #12 Easy Alkaline Lemonade Smoothie

This smoothie is just perfect on a hot summer day. It will help you stay refreshed and energized. No need to drink soda or artificially processed drinks.

Hydrate yourself properly and mindfully and give your body what it needs to thrive.

Serves: 2-3
Ingredients
- 2 small lemons, peeled and cut into smaller pieces
- 2 tablespoons chia seeds
- 2 cups almond milk, unsweetened
- 1 teaspoon cinnamon powder
- 1 cup ice cubes
- Stevia to sweeten, if needed

Instructions
1. Place everything in a blender.
2. Process until smooth.
3. Serve chilled and enjoy! This smoothie also makes a great morning detox drink.

Recipe #13 Full Alkaline Satisfaction Smoothie

Parsley is a highly alkaline forming ingredient, an excellent source of vitamins K and C as well as a good source of vitamin A, and iron.

In this recipe, parsley blends well with sweet potato and zucchini to conjure up an unforgettable alkaline smoothie that can also be served as a quick soup for lunch or dinner.

Serves: 2-3
Ingredients
- Half cup parsley leaves, washed
- 2 cups organic tomato juice
- A handful of almonds, soaked overnight
- 2 big sweet potatoes, cooked and peeled
- 1 small zucchini, peeled and slightly cooked or steamed
- A pinch of Himalayan salt
- A pinch of black pepper

Instructions
1. Place all the ingredients in a blender.
2. Process well until smooth.
3. Enjoy!

Recipe #14 Sweet Dreams Smoothie

This smoothie is designed to help you relax and sleep better. Enjoy it in the evening and allow your body to refuel while you sleep.

This smoothie is light and creamy, perfect for the evening, but at the same time, it will make you feel full so that you no longer feel like snacking at night.

Serves:1- 2
Ingredients
- 1 cup of chamomile infusion (use 1 teabag per cup), cooled
- 1 cup almond milk
- 1 big sweet potato, peeled and cooked
- A handful or arugula leaves, washed
- 1 pinch of Himalayan salt

Instructions
1. Combine all the ingredients in a blender.
2. Process well until smooth.
3. Serve and enjoy!

Recipe #15 Feel Lighter Herbal Smoothie

This smoothie uses horsetail infusion, a natural remedy aimed at reducing water retention and speeding up detoxification.

Ginger makes this smoothie taste interesting while adding some anti-inflammatory properties too. Grapefruit brings some vitamin C and alkaline minerals to the table, while the coconut milk makes the whole blend nice and creamy.

Serves: 2
Ingredients
- 1 cup horsetail infusion, cooled down (use 1 tea bag per cup)
- 1 cup coconut milk
- 2 grapefruits, peeled and cut into smaller pieces
- 1-inch ginger
- 2 tablespoons chia seed powder
- Optional: stevia to sweeten
- Optional: a few ice cubes
- A slice of lime to serve

Instructions
1. Blend all the ingredients in a blender.
2. Serve in a smoothie glass and garnish with a slice of lime.
3. If needed, sweeten with stevia and add some ice cubes for optimal refreshment.

Recipe #16 Creamy Green Smoothie

This is another example of a simple, alkaline smoothie that can also be served as a nourishing raw soup.

Cucumbers are real alkaline super foods that are very often overlooked. Yet, they offer both vitamin C and vitamin A as well as alkaline minerals such as magnesium, potassium and manganese.

Arugula adds a nice, slightly spicy taste and makes this smoothie a proper green smoothie.

Serves: 1-2
Ingredients
- 2 big cucumbers, peeled and sliced
- 1 cup fresh arugula leaves
- 1 clove garlic, peeled
- 1 cup coconut milk or almond milk, unsweetened
- A few slices of avocado
- 1 tablespoon hemp seed protein powder
- 1 tablespoon chia seed powder
- Pinch of black pepper
- Pinch of Himalayan salt
- A small handful of fresh cilantro leaves to garnish

Instructions
1. Place in a blender and process until smooth.
2. Serve in a smoothie glass as a smoothie, or in a small soup bowl. Garnish with fresh cilantro.

Recipe #17 Easy Ginger Turmeric Anti-Inflammatory Smoothie

This smoothie is an excellent natural remedy to boost your immune system. It's simple and effective. I always try to enrich my diet with ginger and turmeric, so using them in my smoothies is one of the best ways to make sure I get those simple superfoods into my diet.

When peeling turmeric, I recommend you use gloves, otherwise you will end up with funky orange nails and hands for the next day or two.

Serves: 1-2
Ingredients
- 2-inches ginger, washed and peeled
- 2-inches turmeric, washed and peeled
- 1 big cucumber, peeled and chopped
- Half an avocado, pitted
- A few lemon slices, peeled
- 1 cup coconut water
- A few ice cubes
- Himalayan salt to taste

Instructions
1. Place everything in a blender and process until smooth.
2. Serve in a smoothie glass, add some more ice cubes if needed and enjoy.

Recipe #18 Sweet Herbal Mint Smoothie

Fennel tea is one of my favorite herbal teas. It helps alleviate anxiety, makes you sleep better and helps stimulate metabolism as well as fight off colds and flu.

It tastes delicious in a smoothie when combined with naturally creamy, plant-based milk. For example, almond milk and some healthy, alkaline fruits.

Serves: 1-2
Ingredients
- 1 cup fennel tea (use 1 fennel tea bag per 1 cup of boiling water), cooled down
- Half cup almond milk, unsweetened
- 1 grapefruit, peeled and cut into smaller pieces
- Half avocado, peeled and pitted
- 1-inch ginger, peeled
- A few mint leaves to garnish
- A few ice cubes to serve
- Optional: stevia to sweeten

Instructions
1. Place all the ingredients in a blender.
2. Process well until smooth.
   Pour into a smoothie glass and serve with some ice cubes and fresh mint leaves. Enjoy!

Recipe #19 Creamy Antioxidant Rooibos Smoothie

Rooibos is considered an alkaline tea, because of its high mineral and antioxidant content. In fact, it's one of my favorite teas, and it appears quite often in my recipes, especially in my book *Alkaline Teas*.

It blends well with ginger, turmeric and refreshing, vitamin C-packed grapefruit.

Serves: 2

Ingredients

- 1 cup of rooibos tea, cooled down (use 1 teabag per cup)
- Half cup almond or coconut milk
- 1 inch ginger, peeled
- 1 -inch turmeric, peeled (orange nails- remember to get kitchen gloves...)
- 1 big grapefruit, peeled and cut into smaller chunks
- A handful of almonds, raw and soaked in water for at least a few hours
- A few lime or lemon slices to garnish

Instructions

1. Place all the ingredients in a blender.
2. Process well until smooth.
3. Pour into a smoothie glass and garnish with some lime or lemon slices.
4. Enjoy!

Optional- if needed, sweeten with stevia.

If you enjoy rooibos tea in your smoothies, make sure you always have some in your fridge so that it's ready to grab to make a mineral rich alkaline smoothie to help you stay energized naturally. It's also a great tool to help you drink less coffee and enjoy more of a caffeine-free, naturally energized lifestyle.

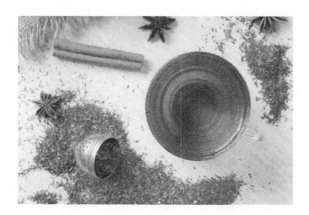

Recipe #20 Irresistible Spicy Green Veggie Smoothie

What I really love about veggie smoothies is that they can also be turned into quick, nourishing soups (raw or lightly cooked).

I very often get asked how to put all those veggies together.

Well, vegetable smoothies always work well. To make them taste amazing, all we need are some herbs and spices.

Serves: 2-3
Ingredients
- A few broccoli florets, raw or steamed
- 1 big zucchini, peeled, raw or steamed
- 1 cup artichoke hearts, cooked
- 2 cups coconut milk, thick, unsweetened
- A generous pinch of Himalayan salt
- 1 tablespoon chia seeds
- 2 garlic cloves, peeled
- A pinch of black pepper
- A pinch of chili powder
- A pinch of curry powder
- Optional: A few cilantro leaves to garnish
- Optional: 2 tablespoons chopped chives to garnish
- Some filtered, preferably alkaline, water if needed to experiment with consistency

Instructions

1. Place all the ingredients in a blender.
2. Process until smooth.
3. If needed, add some water and process again.
4. Serve in a smoothie glass or a small soup bowl.
5. Sprinkle over some cilantro and chives.
6. Enjoy!

Recipe #21 Red Balance Spicy Smoothie

Tomatoes and red bell peppers blend well together while creating a true superfood smoothie. The best part? You don't need any weird exotic foods. All the ingredients are easily obtainable.

Garlic and ginger add to the anti-inflammatory and immune system boosting properties of this smoothie. Oh, and if you want, you can serve this smoothie as a delicious raw, or almost raw, soup. Perfect for a hot summer day when you don't feel like cooking.

Serves: 2
Ingredients
- 2 red bell peppers, chopped
- 4 tomatoes, cut into smaller pieces
- 1 cup water, filtered, preferably alkaline
- 1 small garlic clove, peeled
- 2 inches ginger, peeled
- 1 tablespoon hemp seed protein powder
- 1 tablespoon avocado or olive oil
- Pinch of Himalayan salt to taste
- Pinch of black pepper to taste
- Optional: 2 tablespoons chopped chives to garnish

Instructions
1. Blend all the ingredients in a blender or a food processor.
2. If needed, add more water.
3. Serve in a smoothie glass or a small soup bowl and garnish with some chives. Enjoy!

Recipe #22 Super Alkaline Treat Smoothie

This smoothie is a healthy, natural treat you can turn to whenever you are craving something sweet. Its good fats and natural protein from almonds will keep you full for hours.

Serves: 1-2
Ingredients
- 1 cup thick coconut milk, unsweetened
- 1 tablespoon coconut oil
- A big handful of almonds, soaked in water for at least a few hours
- 1 teaspoon cinnamon powder
- Half teaspoon maca powder
- 2 tablespoons chia seeds
- Optional: stevia to sweeten

Instructions
1. Place all the ingredients in a blender.
2. Process well until smooth.
3. If needed, sweeten with stevia.
4. Chill in a fridge for a few hours.
5. Serve in a smoothie glass or a dessert bowl, with a spoon.

Recipe #23 Deep Relaxation Holistic Smoothie

Ashwagandha is known as an adaptogenic herb. Adaptogens are substances such as amino acids, vitamins and herbs that modulate the body's response to stress and/or a changing environment, both of which are consistent aspects of modern-day life.

Adaptogens are known to help the body cope with and fight against external stressors such as toxins and the environment, as well as internal stressors such as anxiety and insomnia and depression.

Serves: 1-2
Ingredients
- 2 small carrots, peeled
- 1 cup almond milk
- 1 tablespoon chia seeds
- Half avocado, peeled and pitted
- A handful of shredded coconut
- Half teaspoon Ashwagandha powder

Instructions
1. Blend everything together until smooth.
2. Serve in a smoothie glass and enjoy!

Recipe #24 Alkaline Keto Gazpacho Smoothie

This smoothie combines the Mediterranean taste of refreshing Spanish gazpacho with good fats, chlorophyll-rich, healing greens and natural protein. It's tasty, nourishing and very easy to make.

Serves: 2
Ingredients

- 2 medium sized cucumbers, peeled and chopped
- 1 big garlic clove, peeled
- 1 tablespoon extra-virgin, cold pressed olive oil
- 1 avocado, peeled and pitted
- A handful of fresh spinach
- A handful of raw cashews, soaked in water for at least a few hours
- 1 cup water, filtered, preferably alkaline
- Pinch of Himalayan salt
- Pinch of black pepper

Instructions

1. Place all the ingredients in a blender and process until smooth.
2. Serve in a smoothie glass or a small soup bowl.
3. Enjoy!

Recipe #25 Leafy Leaf Powerhouse Detox Smoothie

Celery is rich in vitamin C, fiber, alkaline minerals such as potassium and is also very hydrating and replenishing.

Whenever I buy celery, I like to use its leaves to add to my smoothies and keep celery sticks to snack on with some hummus or guacamole (yes, I should probably write a book on alkaline snacks).

This smoothie combines the best of the almighty, chlorophyll rich greens to help your body nourish and refuel so that you can enjoy optimal energy.

Serves: 2-3
Ingredients
- A small handful of celery leaves
- A small handful of cilantro leaves (+ a few extra to garnish)
- A small handful of spinach leaves
- A small handful or parsley leaves
- A small handful of kale leaves
- A few fresh mint leaves
- 2 cups almond or coconut milk
- 1 tablespoon of flax seed or avocado oil
- Himalayan salt and black pepper to taste

Instructions
1. Place all the ingredients in a blender and process until smooth.
2. Season with Himalayan salt and black pepper.

3. Serve in a smoothie bowl or glass and garnish with some fresh cilantro leaves.

Recipes #26- #50

Balanced Alkaline Smoothies

The following smoothie recipes follow the 80-20 alkaline rule.

They are still super rich in alkaline foods; however, they also use other ingredients to create more taste and balance to help you make a variety of healthy, smoothies you will never get bored with.

They may also be easier to get started on for alkaline beginners, or for people interested in exploring different, healthy ways of making smoothies.

Recipe #26 Lime Chlorophyll Energy Smoothie

Not only is this alkaline smoothie rich in protein and chlorophyll, but it will also help you boost your immune system by enriching your diet with vitamin C and a myriad of alkaline minerals.

Perfect on a hot summer day when hydration and balance should be our number one priority.

Serves: 1-2
Ingredients
- 2 big limes, peeled
- Half cup water, filtered, preferably alkaline
- Half cup coconut water
- A handful of kale leaves, washed
- A handful of cashews, soaked in water for at least a few hours
- 1 teaspoon cinnamon powder
- 1 small banana, peeled
- A generous pinch of nutmeg
- 1 lime wedge to garnish (1 per serving)

Instructions
1. Place in a blender.
2. Process until smooth.
3. Serve in a smoothie glass and garnish with a wedge of lime. Enjoy!

Recipe #27 Arugula Almond Smoothie Express

I always say that simplicity is wellness. On busy days, it's good to have a simple, staple recipe you can make in less than two minutes.

With this recipe, you get two generous servings of greens, natural protein and good fats to help you stay energized. Make it, drink it and forget it.

Serves: 1-2
Ingredients
- 2 handfuls of arugula leaves
- 1 cup almond milk
- 1 green apple, peeled
- 1 tablespoon coconut oil

Instructions
1. Place all the ingredients in a blender.
2. Process until smooth.
3. Enjoy!

Recipe #28 Simple Vanilla Alkaline Smoothie

This smoothie uses pomegranate, which is a naturally alkaline fruit that is rich in nutrients and super-low in sugar. Shredded coconut and vanilla bring in an amazing aroma and taste. Blueberries add in natural antioxidants and an amazing taste.

Serves: 1-2

Ingredients
- 1 cup cashew milk or gluten free oat milk
- A handful of shredded coconut
- Half cup pomegranate
- Half cup blueberries
- Half teaspoon vanilla powder
- Half teaspoon moringa powder
- A few mint leaves

Instructions
1. Place all the ingredients in a blender.
2. Process until smooth.
3. Serve in a smoothie glass and enjoy!

Recipe #29 Delicious Hydration Smoothie

Watercress is a very alkaline green ingredient, rich in vitamin A, C, K as well as magnesium and potassium.

In this smoothie, it teams up with watermelon to create an amazing, refreshing smoothie, perfect for a hot summer day or after working out.

Serves: 1-2
Ingredients
- 1 cup watermelon chunks
- 1 cup watercress
- 1 cup coconut water
- Half teaspoon moringa green powder (optional)
- A few mint leaves
- A few ice cubes

Instructions
1. Place all the ingredients in a blender.
2. Process until smooth.
3. Serve in a smoothie glass, well chilled.
4. Enjoy! Nothing feels better than using your smoothies to sneak some greens into your diet.

Recipe #30 Super Antioxidant Smoothie

This smoothie can also be served as quick smoothie bowl, with some nuts and seeds.

It makes a great, nutritious, alkaline-based breakfast, rich in good protein and healthy antioxidants.

Serves: 1-2
Ingredients
- 1 cup of fresh dairy-free vegan yogurt (for example almond or coconut)
- Half an avocado, peeled and pitted
- Half cup blueberries, washed
- Half teaspoon green powder of your choice
- A handful of raw cashews, soaked in water for at least a few hours
- A pinch of cinnamon powder to serve

Instructions
1. Place all the ingredients in a blender.
2. Process until smooth.
3. Serve in a bowl or a smoothie glass and sprinkle over some cinnamon powder.
4. Enjoy!

Recipe #31 Oil Yourself UP Sweet Protein Smoothie

This recipe uses hemp oil, which is great to re-balance hormones, soothe anxiety and improve the mood.

The delicious blend of refreshing greens, fruit and dates makes it a real treat and a comforting smoothie.

Serves: 1-2
Ingredients
- Half cup strawberries, well washed
- 1 tablespoon hemp oil
- 1 cup oat milk, gluten-free, no added sugar
- A handful of cilantro leaves, well washed
- A handful of mint leaves, washed
- A few dates, pitted

Instructions
1. Place all the ingredients in a blender.
2. Process until smooth.
3. Serve in a smoothie glass, or a bowl and enjoy!

Recipe #32 Blueberry Mint Dream

This is a simple herbal smoothie antioxidant recipe that is great for digestion and relaxation.

It's also a smart way to sneak in some greens.

Serves: 1-2
Ingredients
- Half cup blueberries, washed
- Half avocado, peeled and pitted
- A handful of baby spinach leaves, washed
- A few mint leaves, washed
- A few banana slices
- Half teaspoon of fresh vanilla powder
- Half teaspoon of cinnamon powder
- Half cup almond milk
- 1 cup chamomile infusion, cooled down (use 1 teabag per cup)

Instructions
1. Place almond milk, mint leaves and vanilla in a blender.
2. Process until smooth.
3. Pour into a smoothie glass and mix it with chamomile infusion.
4. Enjoy!

Recipe #33 Energizing Orange Smoothie

Good fats from avocado and coconut oil will help you stay full for longer. They also prevent sugar cravings.

Oranges bring some vitamin C to the table and make the smoothie taste delicious.

Moringa powder is a highly alkalizing, anti-inflammatory and antioxidant ingredient. It's rich in calcium and phosphorous to help you have strong bones.

Serves: 1-2
Ingredients
- 1 tablespoon coconut oil
- 1 cup of hazelnut or other nut milk of your choice
- 1 big orange, peeled and cut into smaller pieces
- A handful of arugula leaves or spinach leaves
- Half avocado, peeled and pitted
- 1 teaspoon moringa powder

Instructions
1. Place all the ingredients in a blender.
2. Process until smooth.
3. Pour into a smoothie glass, stir well, serve and enjoy!

Recipe #34 Colorful Anti-Inflammatory Smoothie

This smoothie has a beautiful orange color.
It tastes delicious and uses some alkaline superfoods such as turmeric and ginger.

Peaches and apricots make this smoothie taste amazing.

Serves: 2-3
Ingredients
- 2 small peaches, pitted
- A handful of dried apricots, no added sugar
- 1 cup water, filtered, preferably alkaline
- 1-inch ginger peeled
- 1-inch turmeric peeled
- 1 teaspoon cinnamon powder

Instructions
1. Place all the ingredients in a blender.
2. Process until smooth.
3. Serve in a smoothie glass or a bowl.

Recipe #35 Almond and Flaxseed Green Protein Smoothie

The flaxseed meal is an excellent source of Omega-3 fatty acids, aka "good fats".

Good fats are also found in almonds, so this smoothie is packed full of both healthy fats and protein.

After having this smoothie, not only will you feel full and satisfied but you will also get an energy boost.

Serves: 1-2
Ingredients
- 1 big green apple, peeled
- 2 dates, pitted
- 1 cup of almond milk
- 2 teaspoons of flaxseed meal
- A handful of fresh baby spinach, washed
- Optional: coconut water, or filtered, alkaline water for thinner consistency, if preferred

Instructions
1. Place all ingredients in a blender.
2. Blend well.
3. If needed, add more water and blend again.
4. Serve into a chilled glass and enjoy!

Recipe #36 Spicy Mediterranean Smoothie with Olives

This smoothie is an excellent energy boosting smoothie full of alkaline vegetables and greens.

It's also very tasty as it uses olives and spices.

Serves: 3-4
Ingredients
- A handful of fresh arugula leaves, washed
- 1 small red bell pepper, chopped
- 1 small green bell pepper, chopped
- 1 cup almond milk
- 1 cup water, filtered, preferably alkaline
- A handful of raw cashews, soaked in water for at least a few hours
- Himalayan salt to taste
- A pinch of oregano
- 1 garlic clove, peeled
- A pinch of hot chili powder
- Half cup green olives, pitted
- 2 tablespoons of apple cider vinegar

Instructions
1. Place all the ingredients in a blender.
2. Process well until smooth.
3. Serve and enjoy!

   Suggestion – you can serve the olives on top of this "smoothie soup" instead of blending them in.

Recipe #37 The Green Factory Smoothie

Spinach is packed with iron. Watercress is the leader of anti-aging vegetables, with enormous amounts of vitamin K and other healthy nutrients that contribute to healthy skin, hair and nails.

We are also adding oranges here, for their vitamin C and natural sweetness.

Serves: 2-3
Ingredients
- Half cup of spinach
- Half cup of watercress
- 2 oranges, peeled and cut into smaller pieces
- 1 cup of any nut milk of your choice
- 1 tablespoon coconut oil
- 1 tablespoon hemp seed powder
- 1 tablespoon cocoa powder

Instructions
1. Add all ingredients to a high-powered blender and processed until smooth.
2. Serve and enjoy!

Recipe #38 Broccoli Power Smoothie

We all know that broccoli is good for us, but getting it into our diets can present a challenge. That is why I started adding it into my smoothies- so much easier!

A few raw broccoli florets here and there can really compound to amazing results.

Serves: 1-2

Ingredients

- A few raw broccoli florets
- 1 big orange, peeled
- 1 cup of almond milk
- 2 tablespoons of organic almond butter
- Half teaspoon of nutmeg powder
- 1 tablespoon hemp seeds
- A few walnuts, soaked in water for at least a few hours

Instructions

1. Add all ingredients to a blender.
2. Process until well combined.
3. Pour into a glass and serve.

Recipe #39 Protein Superfood Treat Smoothie

This superfood smoothie is highly nutritious. It focuses mostly on alkaline ingredients like avocado, sweet potato, coconut milk and flaxseed.

To add some variety, it also uses cocoa powder (great natural mood enhancer) and blueberries. This is a perfect healthy smoothie that you can enjoy as a treat.

Serves:1-2
Ingredients
- 1 cup coconut milk
- Half cup water, filtered, preferably alkaline
- 1 sweet potato, peeled and cooked
- Half avocado, peeled and pitted
- 2 tablespoons of flaxseed meal
- 1 tablespoon cocoa powder
- Half cup blueberries
- 1 teaspoon vanilla extract

Instructions
1. Put all the ingredients into a blender.
2. Blend well until smooth.
3. Pour into a chilled glass.
4. Serve and enjoy!

Recipe#40 Green Refreshment Mineral Smoothie

This smoothie offers a balanced mix of fruits and veggies as well as natural protein and good fats.

Coconut water makes this smoothie naturally sweet and adds in a ton of nutrients such as vitamin C, magnesium, manganese, potassium and calcium.

Serves: 1-2
Ingredients
- Half cup pineapple chunks
- Half cup arugula leaves, washed
- 1 small lime, peeled
- 1 big cucumber, peeled and cut into smaller pieces
- A handful of fresh mint, washed
- 1 tablespoon chia seeds
- 1 tablespoon almonds, soaked in water for at least a few hours
- 1 cup coconut water

Instructions
1. Put all ingredients into a blender.
2. Process well until smooth.
3. If needed, add more water and blend again.
4. Pour into a chilled glass and serve.

Recipe #41 Green Coconut Smoothie

This smoothie is a perfectly nutritious, moderately alkaline smoothie to enjoy first thing in the morning.

Green tea can be added if you need a quick energy boost. While it's not considered alkaline (the alkaline lifestyle prefers a caffeine-free option), it's still a true superfood ingredient full of antioxidants.

The energy boost it provides is more sustainable than coffee, especially if you combine it with other nutritious ingredients like in this smoothie. It can be a great "transition smoothie", if you would like to reduce your coffee intake without experiencing nasty withdrawal symptoms.

Servings: 2
Ingredients
- 1 cup green tea, cooled down (use 1 tea bag per cup)
- Half cup coconut milk
- 2 green apples, peeled, and cut into smaller pieces
- A few avocado slices
- A handful of mint leaves, washed
- Optional – stevia to sweeten

Instructions
1. Place all the ingredients in a blender.
2. Process until smooth.
3. If needed, add a bit more water or coconut milk.
4. Enjoy!

Recipe #42 Cinnamon Sweetness Smoothie

This smoothie is a great recipe for "recycling" some broccoli leftovers. Oranges and cinnamon make this smoothie naturally sweet and yummy. Almond milk adds to the creaminess and provides natural protein, boosted by the chia seeds.

If you don't know how to get more broccoli into your diet, or don't like cooked broccoli in meals, then this smoothie will help!

Servings: 2
Ingredients
- A few broccoli florets, raw or steamed
- 2 small oranges, peeled and cut into smaller pieces
- 1 cup almond milk
- 1 teaspoon cinnamon powder
- 1 tablespoon chia seeds

Instructions
1. Blend all the ingredients.
2. If needed, add more water or any plant-based milk of your choice.
3. Pour into a glass and enjoy.

Recipe #43 Red Tea Horsetail Fat Burn Smoothie

This recipe is another moderately alkaline smoothie that calls for a little bit of red tea, well known for its fat-burning properties.

It blends well with alkaline horsetail infusion- a natural remedy to ease water retention symptoms and help you feel lighter (great for the summer or if you spend lots of time in sitting or standing jobs).

Grapefruit and ginger add to the alkaline side of this smoothie and watermelon creates balance and natural sweetness that makes this smoothie so refreshing and delicious.

Servings: 2
Ingredients
- 2 grapefruits, peeled and cut into smaller pieces
- 1-inch ginger, peeled
- 1 cup watermelon chunks
- 1 cup horsetail infusion, cooled down (use 1 teabag per cup)
- 1 cup red tea (use 1 teabag per cup)
- Ice cubes
- Mint leaves to garnish

Instructions
1. Blend all the ingredients using a blender or a food processor.
2. Pour into a glass or a bowl.
3. Add in some mint leaves and ice cubes.
4. Enjoy!

Recipe #44 Hormone Rebalancer Smoothie

This smoothie recipe is a fantastic option if you want to take a break from traditional leafy green smoothies, but you still want to experience all the health benefits of smoothies rich in protein and alkaline foods.

This recipe is another balanced, moderately alkaline smoothie, that uses a bit of kiwi for natural sweetness and a ton of vitamin C. Maca is a great superfood, well known for its natural, energy boosting properties and hormone balancing for women.

Servings: 1-2
Ingredients
- 1 big grapefruit, peeled and halved
- 1 kiwi, peeled
- 1 cup coconut water
- 1 inch ginger, peeled
- 1 tablespoon coconut oil
- Half teaspoon maca powder

Instructions
1. Blend all the ingredients in a blender.
2. Serve and enjoy!

Recipe #45 Delicious Smoothie Soup

This moderately alkaline recipe can be used both as a smoothie and a soup. It focuses on healthy, natural plant-based fats and hydrating veggies. Green and black olives make this smoothie taste delicious!

Servings: 1-2
Ingredients
- 1 big cucumber, peeled
- 1 small avocado, peeled and pitted
- A handful cilantro leaves, washed
- 1 cup cashew milk, unsweetened, unsalted
- A handful of raw cashews, soaked in water for at least a few hours
- A handful of green olives
- A handful of black olives
- 2 tablespoons apple cider vinegar
- Himalayan salt and black pepper to taste

Instructions
1. Blend all the ingredients in a blender.
2. Serve in a smoothie glass or in a small soup bowl.
3. Enjoy!

Most alkaline experts agree that fermented foods, like olives, are not alkaline forming. Neither are vinegars. However, these foods, even though not in the alkaline category, do offer a myriad of other health benefits.

While alkalinity is one of the crucial factors for maintaining our health and wellbeing, there are many other health foods (not necessarily alkaline) that we can experiment with (as a part of 80/20 rule).

So, I don't use ACV (apple cider vinegar) for strictly alkaline purposes, but I like to add a bit to my salads, soups and smoothies, just to enjoy more variety with my recipes. I also use ACV for cleaning.

Olives are one of my favorite non-alkaline foods. They are a fantastically healthy snack, naturally rich in good fats and gut-friendly bacteria.

Recipe #46 Creamy Veggie Smoothie

This recipe uses healing alkaline veggies like cauliflower, and, at the same time, adds in some garlic to help you strengthen your immune system.

Cashew milk and cashew nuts make this recipe very creamy and add protein. Olives and a bit of apple cider vinegar add to the smoothie's original taste.

Servings: 1-2
Ingredients
- 1 cup cauliflower florets, lightly cooked or steamed, cut into smaller pieces
- 1 cup thick cashew milk
- A handful of cashews, soaked in water for at least a few hours
- 1 tablespoon avocado oil
- 2 garlic cloves, peeled and minced
- A handful of spicy green olives, pitted
- 1 tablespoon apple cider vinegar
- Himalayan salt to taste

Instructions
1. Blend all the ingredients in a blender until smooth.
2. If needed, add more water.
3. Serve as a smoothie, or a "smoothie soup".
4. Enjoy!

Recipe # 47 Simple Anti-Inflammatory Smoothie

This smoothie is perfect if your goal is to have more energy and reduce inflammation.

It focuses on two highly anti-inflammatory ingredients- turmeric and ginger. Fresh almond milk is very alkalizing and rich in natural protein. Good fats will help you stay full and focused for hours.

Apple adds healthy fiber and makes this moderately alkaline smoothie taste amazing.

Serves: 1-2
Ingredients
- Half cup fresh almond milk, unsweetened
- Half cup water, filtered, preferably alkaline water
- 1 green apple, sliced, seeds removed
- 2-inches ginger, peeled
- 2-inches turmeric, peeled
- 1 tablespoon avocado oil

Instructions
1. Blend all the ingredients until smooth.
2. Serve and enjoy!

Recipe #48 Green Balance Energy Smoothie

This delicious moderately alkaline smoothie combines the best of the chlorophyll rich greens with the freshness and sweetness of melon.

It also uses spirulina, a blue-green algae powder that adds in a ton of nutrients such as calcium, magnesium and potassium as well as protein.

Serves: 3
Ingredients
- 1 cup coconut milk, unsweetened
- 1 cup water, filtered, preferably alkaline
- A handful of fresh spinach leaves, washed
- A handful of watercress, washed
- A handful of arugula leaves, washed
- 1 cup melon chunks
- 1 teaspoon spirulina powder

+ a few lime slices and ice cubes to serve if needed

Instructions
1. Place all the ingredients in a blender.
2. Process until smooth.
3. Serve and enjoy!
4. This smoothie tastes delicious when chilled or half frozen.

Recipe #55 Not So Alkaline Banana Dream

This recipe is simple, delicious and nutritious, rich in good protein, fats and healthy carbohydrates as well as magnesium.

It's great to enjoy chilled, after hiking or working out. Banana and lemons blend well together, creating a nice balance of taste, and natural "creaminess".

Serves: 1-2
Ingredients
- 1 big banana
- 1 big lemon
- 1 cup coconut or almond milk
- 1 teaspoon chia seeds
- 1 teaspoon nutritional yeast

Instructions
1. Blend all the ingredients until smooth.
2. Serve and enjoy!

Bonus Recipes- Delicious Alkaline Smoothie Bowl Recipes

The following bonus recipes will inspire you to start turning some of your smoothies into delicious and creative smoothie bowls.

Smoothie bowls are amazing as a quick breakfast or a guilt-free snack. They can be sweet or sour.

They will help you add a ton of healing superfoods as well as alkaline foods into your diet.

Enjoy!

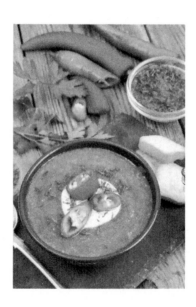

Bonus Recipe #1 Anti-Inflammatory Smoothie Bowl

This smoothie offers a unique combination of vitamin C and anti-inflammatory, highly alkalizing ingredients like ginger and turmeric. It's especially recommended for winter and fall because it helps boost the immune system to prevent flu and colds.

If you dread the idea of including raw spinach leaves in your smoothie bowl, have no fear. Spinach and oranges are an excellent combo, not only because orange will help neutralize the taste of the spinach, but also because the vitamin C from the oranges (or any other vitamin C-rich foods, I am not saying it must be oranges) helps in iron absorption.

Serves: 1-2
Ingredients for the Smoothie
- A handful of fresh spinach leaves
- 1 orange, peeled
- 1 one-inch piece of ginger root, peeled
- half teaspoon turmeric
- 1 cup coconut milk

More Ingredients for the Toppings:
- Handful of blueberries
- A few fresh mint leaves
- 2 tablespoons crushed almonds or almond powder

Instructions

1. Blend all the ingredients until smooth. If you are making this smoothie on a hot summer day, feel free to add some ice cubes. Pour into a bowl.
2. Add the rest of the ingredients on top.
3. You can enjoy your smoothie bowl now or store it in the fridge for later.

Bonus Recipe #2 From the Sea Bowl

Another option for a not-so-sweet smoothie. It offers a myriad of nutrients such as B vitamins and iodine from nori and Omega-3s from chia seeds.

With some green veggies like zucchini and kale, you are bound to feel energized the way you deserve.

Serves: 1-2
Ingredients
- 2 nori sheets, soaked in water
- 1 cup coconut milk
- Half avocado, peeled and pitted
- 1 small zucchini, peeled and chopped, raw or steamed
- Handful of kale (thick stalks removed)
- 1 teaspoon flax seeds
- 1 teaspoon chia seeds
- 1 tablespoon almond butter
- 1 tablespoon ground almonds
- Himalayan salt to taste

More Ingredients for the Toppings
- Handful of pistachios
- Handful of crushed cashews
- 1 slice of lemon

Instructions

1. Blend all the ingredients until smooth. If you are making this smoothie on a hot summer day, feel free to add some ice cubes. Pour into a bowl.
2. Mix in the rest of the ingredients by placing them on top. Enjoy!

Bonus Recipe #3 Super Energy Creamy Smoothie Bowl

This is an incredible smoothie with a creamy consistency and energizing ingredients. It's perfect for moments of mental and physical stress.

Maca is an amazing hormone balancer, particularly for women. Cinnamon and cacao are great mood boosters and add to the feeling of comfort and coziness.

Serves: 1-2
Ingredients for the Smoothie
- 1 cup hazelnut milk
- 1 teaspoon maca powder
- 1 teaspoon raw cacao powder
- 1 avocado, peeled and pitted
- Half teaspoon cinnamon
- Handful of ice (optional)
- Half tablespoon coconut oil

More Ingredients for the Toppings
- 2 tablespoons of coconut cream or coconut yogurt
- Handful of blueberries
- 2 slices of lime

Instructions
1. Blend all the ingredients until smooth. If you are making this smoothie on a hot summer day, feel free to add some ice cubes. Pour into a bowl.

2. Mix in the rest of the ingredients. First, sprinkle the coconut cream or yogurt on top of the smoothie and then top it with blueberries and garnish with lime slices.

3. You can enjoy your smoothie bowl now or store it in the fridge for later.

Bonus Recipe #4 Super Green Bowl

Chlorophyll is the secret power of alkalinity. All you need to do is create a habit of adding a few drops of liquid chlorophyll to your smoothie bowls.

You can also use powdered chlorophyll or even green powder mix that contains different alkaline herbs.

Serves: 1-2
Ingredients
- A handful of baby spinach leaves
- 4 tablespoons fresh mint leaves
- 1 cup coconut milk
- 1 teaspoon chlorophyll powder (or a few drops of liquid chlorophyll), or 1 teaspoon of any other green powder
- A handful of blueberries
- Half an apple

More Ingredients for the Toppings
- Handful of sunflower seeds
- Handful of hemp seeds
- 1 slice of lemon or lime
- A few dates (pitted) or raisins
- A few grapes

Instructions

1. Blend all the ingredients until smooth. If you are making this smoothie on a hot summer day, feel free to add some ice cubes. Pour into a bowl.
2. Mix in the rest of the ingredients by placing them on top.
3. You can enjoy your smoothie bowl now or store it in the fridge for later.

Bonus Recipe #5 Sweet Potato Alkaline Smoothie Bowl

Many people fear carbohydrates, but when it comes to healthy carbs, there is nothing to fear.

They will help you start the day feeling energized and happy. This is also a fantastic pre-workout recipe where sweet potatoes are the primary ingredient.

With some added omega-3 and protein from the flax seeds and green super-alkaline ingredients, you will have an incredible and tasty breakfast or snack.

Serves: 1-2
Ingredients
- 1 cup cooked sweet potatoes, peeled and chopped
- 1 cup of almond or coconut milk (unsweetened)
- Half teaspoon nutmeg
- Half teaspoon ground cinnamon
- 1 teaspoon flax seed
- One small avocado, peeled and pitted
- A few spinach leaves
- Optional: Half teaspoon moringa powder

More Ingredients for the Toppings
- Handful of crushed almonds
- Handful of crushed cashews
- 3 tablespoons fresh orange juice

Instructions

1. Blend all the ingredients until smooth. If you are making this smoothie on a hot summer day, feel free to add some ice cubes.
2. Mix in the rest of the ingredients by placing them on top.
3. You can enjoy your smoothie bowl now or store it in the fridge for later.

Bonus Recipe #6 Creamy Guilt-Free Protein Bowl

In this smoothie bowl, not only will you get protein, but also taste, alkalinity, and energy.

Serves: 1-2
Ingredients
- 1 cup frozen raspberries (keep a few for decoration)
- 1 cup coconut yogurt (natural, no added sugar). You can also use coconut cream or thick coconut milk. If you are allergic to coconut or dairy, any plant-based yoghurt will do here, so don't worry.
- 1 tablespoon chia seeds
- A handful of baby spinach
- 1 orange
- 1 small avocado

More Ingredients for the Toppings
- Handful of crushed almonds
- Handful or grapes
- 2 tablespoons almond or coconut powder

Instructions
1. Blend all the ingredients until smooth. If you are making this smoothie on a hot summer day, feel free to add some ice cubes.
2. Mix in the rest of the ingredients by placing them on top.
3. You can enjoy your smoothie bowl now or store it in the fridge for later.

Bonus Recipe #7 Mediterranean Anti-Inflammatory Mix

If you like Mediterranean flavors and spices, you will love this. Who said smoothie bowls must be sweet? Also, this one is super alkaline! It is a fantastic lunch idea.

With a creamy, healthy, filling, alkaline avocado base, the flavors are added to with some glorious fresh herbs that bring these vegetables to life.

Serves: 1-2
Ingredients
- 1 avocado, peeled and pitted
- 1 cup coconut milk, unsweetened
- 2 tablespoons mixed herbs like oregano, mint, and parsley
- Juice of 1 lemon
- 3 tomatoes, peeled
- 1 cucumber, peeled and chopped
- 1 tablespoon cashew nut butter
- 10 green olives
- A few spinach leaves

Ingredients for the Toppings
- Handful of pistachios
- Handful of black olives
- 1 slice of lemon
- A few basil leaves

Instructions

1. Blend all the ingredients until smooth. If you are making this smoothie on a hot summer day, feel free to add some ice cubes. Pour into a bowl.
2. Arrange the other ingredients attractively on top.
3. You can enjoy your smoothie bowl now or store it in the fridge for later.

Final Words

I value health more than anything else in life. I know that when I am healthy, and I feel aligned, I create the best version of myself.

That allows me to focus on helping other people to the best of my ability. I can also focus on growing other areas of my life and creating balance.

Now, at thirty-six years old, I feel like I have cracked the code to wellness and wellbeing- on a physical, emotional and mental level. Still, I am on a never-ending quest of learning and practicing which is my biggest passion in life.

One of my health and wellness mentors once told me: *never stop learning, the moment you stop, it all ends*. And the best way to learn is by doing.

But, you see, it wasn't always that way. I have been through lots of pain and suffering due to serious health problems that plagued me for years. Because of that I felt demotivated and every day was a struggle.

Now, looking back at where I was before, I can say that I am feeling grateful for that pain and suffering for numerous reasons. For instance, I can totally relate to the pain, frustration and discomfort that other people are feeling. That allows me to develop a strong sense of empathy and connection so that I can really help people transition to a healthier, happier and more empowered lifestyle. That passion really keeps me going.

Whenever I receive an email from a happy reader who is now on their own unique journey of transformation, I feel forever grateful and inspired.

So, you may be wondering what exactly happened to me. What led me to my transformation and what my health story is. Well, when I was only four years old, I suffered from a severe attack of uveitis.

"Uveitis *(pronounced you-vee-EYE-tis) is inflammation of the uvea — the middle layer of the eye that consists of the iris, ciliary body and choroid.* **Uveitis** *can have many causes, including eye injury and inflammatory diseases."* – from Wikipedia

It's a condition triggered mostly by autoimmune system disorders and manifests as a serious health condition that can even cause blindness.

That was the diagnosis that most doctors would give me back then.

The treatment was brutal. I even remember getting eye injections during that time, as a kid. I also have a very blurry memory of going to stay at an eye clinic that was located on the other side of my country. Of course, my parents would come and visit me as often as they could, but most of their time was spent back in our hometown working very hard to be able to pay for my treatment.

I had been given huge doses of hormone treatments and antibiotics. The doctors were confused, and it seemed like there was no long-term cure. That was back in the eighties in

Poland. Most medicine required for my treatment, was not even available for us there.

However, my parents had the courage to keep investigating and found a functional medicine eye doctor who was able to help me by combining traditional medicines with natural ones. An interesting thing is that now he's over ninety years old and still working and doing great! Enjoying vibrant health and helping other people.

Luckily for us, my dad also happened to have an amazing friend and colleague from the UK. That colleague of his was very helpful as he managed to find the medication that at that time was not available in my native country.

So that was my first exposure to a holistic approach. <u>Combining standard medicine and scientific research with an integrated approach to health, balance and healing.</u>

I always stress that I am not a fan of some woo-woo or people who totally reject doctors and standard medicine. There is a place for everything, and it's not even about what we do but how we do it. There are many medications that literally save people's lives. At the same time, the integrated, natural approach focuses on lifestyle change, prevention and stimulating the body's natural healing responses as a long-term approach to health and healing. Natural methods very often require time, patience, courage and belief and a very big lifestyle change.

So, to finish my story; the treatment with that functional medicine doctor helped me and my eyes were healed.
From there, all the memory I have of that time is of my dad picking me up from the clinic. I went back to my hometown

and started school, and that was when my little brother was born. Life was good again and I was very happy.

As I was leaving that clinic, the doctor told us that the amount of antibiotics and hormones I had been given as a child was something he had never seen before. He said it would take many years to get it all out of my system and that I may be prone to some hormonal imbalances later as I grew up. He also said that any imbalances in my lifestyle may lead to the uveitis manifesting itself again.

I had a normal, peaceful childhood, although I would very often get sick. Same for when I was a teenager. I would be sick several times a year, sometimes even once a month.

But the uveitis did not come back. Until I was twenty-nine. What a nightmare. When I found out about it from my eye doctor, I felt so depressed. All those vague blurred memories from my childhood got back to my adult life.

I managed to find some courage though. Since I was living abroad, I decided to find a functional medicine eye doctor in my local area. *If it doesn't help*, I said to myself, *I will go back to the same clinic in my home country.*

Although... you know, adult life is different, you've got work to do and bills to pay. So, I decided to look for qualified ophthalmologists locally.

At that time, I was already getting into a heathy lifestyle and was making some big changes in my professional life too. After going through lots of stress because of my pretty unfulfilling work at that time and other problems I was facing, I knew I was out of balance. Something was wrong. And that clearly manifested as a disease.

Luckily, I found an amazing international ophthalmologist who also specialized in natural medicine. In fact, she was integrating standard medicine (so necessary to get all the checkups, data, analysis, diagnosis and reliable information) with cleverly designed natural healing.

I followed her treatment and healed my eye in less than three months.

Following her recommendation, I began looking into an anti-inflammatory diet and that led me to discovering the Alkaline Diet, which by now, I am sure you can tell I am passionate about!

Needless to say, though, at first when I came across it, I felt very skeptical about it and thought it was a fad! What? How can lemons be on alkaline food lists? And how can eating more vegetables can help me feel better?

However, I decided to give it a try and started experiencing a positive transformation. It was a journey, and it still is. Every day we get to choose to do something healthy.

Prior to my transformation with the Alkaline Diet, I suffered from another issue that my doctors hadn't been able to help with...That issue was low energy levels and constant allergies. It was affecting my performance at work. I had no idea what to do, no idea what to eat.

I remember that there was a period where I would get back from work between six and seven in the evening and immediately go back to bed. And while in bed I could not enjoy quality sleep either.

Then, the mornings were a nightmare. Alarm clock and overdoing coffee just to keep going. I just felt so much out of balance and I remember feeling very frustrated and confused.

However, after discovering the Alkaline Diet, things began to change. It started off with my medical condition, the uveitis attack. That really motivated me to change my entire lifestyle.

My whole lifestyle, not just food. The way I lived, thought and also my career. I consciously decided to re-design my life in such a way that health would be my highest priority. I also knew this:

After I transform and make myself super-healthy, strong and energized, I will start sharing and teaching the exact process to other people.

It was a process; the changes didn't come overnight. While transitioning to a healthy lifestyle, many of my old friends would laugh at me because I didn't want to drink with them at the bar.

However, that initial holistic health journey also helped me re-align myself with my true-life purpose and meet many other supportive people. Eventually I became blessed with my own little holistic, alkaline community.

Honestly, everyone is at a different place on their journey and judging other people for their choices is like judging myself from ten years ago so I will leave it here.

My focus is now on 100% empowerment.

The work is still in progress. I am not perfect.
I want to show you that everything is a process and that small decisions lead to a compound effect.

Things don't happen *to* us; they happen *for* us.
Empowerment. Courage. Motivation.

We all get started somewhere. Never compare yourself to other people because your journey is truly unique!

Looking back, like I said, I am grateful for what happened *to* me because it actually happened *for* me.

My own health issues led me to seek and master holistic solutions.

I found my answers in an integrated lifestyle and "alkaline inspired", clean food diets.

With vibrant health you can literally do whatever you want, and it will seem like you have more free time, due to increased energy levels.

Yes, some people might say that what you do is weird. It happened to me many times. But guess what? Some people will be inspired.

And that is my intention. I want you to inspire those around you. Help them make heathy choices. Not by preaching but by living and sharing.

So, be a holistic leader in your small community. Trust me-people will love it!

Okay, enough of motivational talk, I guess you must be on fire right now.

You see, the reason behind me writing my books is not to create a plain and boring "how to" book that gets forgotten in your eBook device or on your bookshelf.

My intention is to really inspire you so that you can use it to transform the way you desire to.

Let's finish off this book with my best tips to help you look and feel amazing.

When you combine the following tips with the recipes and empowering mindset from this book, you will be able to dive deep, transform your body and mind and feel amazing.

Here are a few simple guidelines that will help you transition towards a healthy, alkaline lifestyle. These are compatible with different nutritional lifestyles (Gluten Free, Vegetarian, Vegan) and it's totally up to you what you choose to focus on:

Eliminate processed foods from your diet and say "no" to colas and sodas

There are so many additives and preservatives in these foods. They have been known to create hormone imbalances, make you tired, and add to acidity in your body. It's just not natural for humans to consume those conveniently processed foods.

The label may even say "low in calories or low in fat" but it will not help you in your long-term weight loss or health efforts. In order to start losing weight naturally, your body needs foods that are jam-packed with nutrients. Real foods. Living foods.

This, in turn, will help your body maintain its optimal blood pH almost effortlessly.

Add more raw foods to your diet

Focus on adding lots of vegetables and leafy greens as well as fruits that are naturally low in sugar (for example, limes, lemons, grapefruits, avocados, tomatoes, and pomegranates are alkaline forming fruits).

Reduce/eliminate animal products

These are very acid forming. The good news is that there are many plant-based options out there and tons of way to create delicious alkaline-friendly plant-based meals you will love! Whether you want to eat fully plant-based, or almost plant-based, or you simply want to eat more vegetables, it's your decision, so I am not here to preach the exact way you "should" be eating.

But...even by making most of your diet alkaline plant-based, you will begin to feel lighter and more energized. Also, plant-based recipes are creative and inexpensive.

Drink plenty of clean, filtered water

Preferably drink alkaline water or alkaline fruit-infused water (lemons, grapefruits, limes and pomegranates are great for that).

Add more vegetable juices into your diet

These are a great way to give your body more nutrients and alkalinity that will result in more energy, less inflammation and, if desired, natural weight loss.

Vegetable juices are the best shots of health! I have also written a book called *Alkaline Juicing* if you want to give it a try and want to learn how to juice the right way, to enjoy more energy and health.

Reduce/eliminate processed grains, "crappy carbs" as well as yeast (very acid forming).

Personally, I recommend quinoa instead (it's naturally gluten-free), some sweet potatoes or some fresh seasonal fruit.

You can also use gluten-free wraps or make your own bread.

Reduce/eliminate caffeine

Trust me - it will only make you feel sick and tired in the long run and can even lead to adrenal exhaustion or chronic fatigue.

It may seem a bit drastic at first, and yes, I know what you're thinking- there are so many articles out there praising the benefits of caffeine and coffee.

Yes, I am sure there are, as many people build their business around coffee. That is why there must be something out there that promotes it. At the same time, I agree that everything is good for you in moderation.

As long as you have a healthy foundation, you can have coffee as a treat (I do drink coffee occasionally).

There is no reason to be too strict on yourself, just don't rely on caffeine as your main source of energy. Green tea may be helpful too as a transition, but green tea is not caffeine-free either so don't overdo it.

On the other end of the spectrum - green tea is rich in antioxidants and a great part of a balanced diet, so it's not that you have to get paranoid about all kinds of caffeine. <u>Moderation is the key</u>.

Try to observe your body. Personally, I have noticed that quitting my coffee habits (I used to have 2-3 coffees a day) and replacing coffee with natural herbal teas and infusions has really made my energy levels skyrocket.

Now I sleep better, and I get up feeling nice and fresh. I don't need caffeine to keep me awake. I no longer suffer from tension headaches and I feel calmer.

Yes, I do have a cup of coffee as a treat sometimes, usually when I meet with a friend for a chat, but I no longer depend on it. I choose it; it doesn't choose me.

Think about this and how you can apply this simple tip to your life to achieve total wellbeing. Coffee and caffeine in general are very acid-forming.

I recently started using an Ayurvedic herb called Ashwagandha. It is known as an adaptogenic herb and it can help you restore your energy levels naturally (be sure to consult it with your doctor first, just like in the case of any herb, supplement or natural therapy).

I have also written a book called *Alkaline Teas*. It's all about healing, herbal, alkaline friendly infusions that will help you get your energy naturally so that you don't need to depend on caffeine. In this book, I go deeper into no caffeine drinks. Even skipping your normal cup of coffee here and there and going for a nice herbal infusion now and again can really add to your natural energy levels.

Replace cow's milk with almond milk, coconut milk or any other plant-based friendly milk

As you already know, cow's milk is extremely acid forming and personally, I don't think it makes sense for humans to drink milk that is naturally designed for fattening baby calves not humans.

Quitting dairy is one of the best things I have done for myself. I have noticed that even very little milk would cause digestive problems and it was really easy to fix-I quit drinking milk.

The best thing about the alkaline plant-based diet is that you can still have ice cream and other treats- you just make them with no milk/animal products. It's so much healthier and tastier, totally guilt-free.

With this approach, there is no need to go hungry or be deprived.

Don't fear good fats- coconut oil, olive oil, avocado oil etc.

These alkaline oils are good for you and should replace processed margarines, and artery-clogging trans-fats. This is not to say that you can "drink" them freely. Balance is the key.

Use stevia instead of processed sugar and Himalayan salt instead of regular salt

Stevia is sweet but sugar-free and Himalayan salt contains calcium, iron, potassium and magnesium plus it also contains lower amounts of sodium than regular salt.

Add more spices and herbs to your diet- not only do they make your dishes taste amazing, but they also have anti-inflammatory properties and help you detoxify (cilantro, turmeric, and cinnamon are miraculous).

As you can see, the Alkaline Diet is a pretty common-sense clean diet. Nothing is exaggerated. Nothing is too strict. Nothing is too faddish. Eat more living foods and avoid processed foods. Try to eat more plant-based foods (even if you're not fully vegan).

Add regular relaxation techniques to the Alkaline Diet (including yoga, meditation), time spent in nature, adequate sleep and physical activity (we need to sweat out those toxins) and you have a prescription for health.

It's strange to me that there are so many people putting the Alkaline Diet down. However, the general guidelines I have mentioned above are common sense for a healthy lifestyle and I am sure your doctor would agree with it (more natural foods, less processed junk, eat more veggies, drink more water, add more relaxation, reduce/manage stress).

This is the gist of the Alkaline Diet lifestyle. This is what will make you feel fresh and rejuvenated and help you achieve your ideal weight. The problem is that some people are not willing to take those small common-sense steps and are looking for a "secret formula"- something that will magically help them with no effort at all. I am not judging- I have been guilty of it as well. We all have!

The truth is that whatever changes you want to make in your life (this rule applies not only to health) can be hard. Leaving one's comfort zone is difficult, but with time and practice it becomes easy and automatic.

Holistic success is about applying what we already know and using the information to better our lives. This is what I call "the secret formula." <u>Information in action</u>. I always say that I am very open-minded when it comes to different diets. I never claim that what I do is the only path to wellness and health. I prefer to provide you with information and inspiration so that you can create your own way and choose what works for you. Everyone is different.

You need to learn to listen to your body and be good to yourself.

Everyone is different, which is why your alkaline lifestyle will be different to mine. However, many elements remain similar, and it is my hope that this book has given you the tools, recipes and inspiration you need to be successful on your health and wellness quest.

Feel free to come back to this book whenever you need more motivation.

It's all about making consistent progress and about those small daily decisions.

They will help you create what I like to call *empowering alkaline mini habits*. These, when compounded, will help you to transform in a way you never even thought was possible. It will be an amazing experience.

Finally, I need to ask you for a small favor. It will only take a few minutes of your precious time and will be very helpful for me at this stage. All I am asking you for is your honest review on Amazon. Your review, even a short one, can inspire someone else to start living a healthy lifestyle and enjoy the benefits of alkaline protein smoothies.

Let's make this world a happy, healthy and more empowered place.

That collective transformation starts with small baby steps and micro-actions.

Thank you, thank you, thank you. I am really looking forward to reading your review.

Marta

For bonus resources, inspiration & empowerment, to help you on your journey, join my mailing list at:

www.HolisticWellnessProject.com/alkaline

Printed in Great Britain
by Amazon

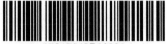

17917048R00081